Ian's account of his journey with his son and family through a major head injury is ongoing. More importantly, it is captured as a whole lived experience, including the explainable, the frightening, the joyful and the mysterious. It is the story before analysis, before explanation and before the extraction of "useful" guidance for professionals that captures the heart. Read the words, see his family and yours and marvel at your good fortune to have this account. Learning will follow.

David A. Gass, MD, CCFP, FCFP
Professor, Department of Family Medicine
Dalhousie University

This is a well written book of compelling nature, capturing attention, giving goosebumps at times, not needing endorsement. We can all identify with it. The anguish and struggle of its characters to be better, to do better, to reach higher is a recipe for ongoing spiritual growth of everyone who is intent on growing and a reminder to those who are missing the opportunity.

Dr. J. N. Vanek, MD, Psychotherapist

Although I am not a health professional, I know only too well as a parent and a journalist that hellish health experiences of the sort experienced by the Powell family can strike at any time—usually when they are utterly unexpected.

Knowing how health care professionals can be expected to respond—one of the lessons of this book—is extremely important knowledge for navigating through the experience.

This book, which could not have been easy to write, involved me in a family's extremely personal emotional experience—and opened my eyes to aspects of Ontario's health system which I have never been exposed to before.

I am grateful to Ian Powell for taking me on the harrowing journey.

Harold Levy.
Criminal lawyer and journalist
Retired as a staff reporter at the
Toronto Star in 2006.

From Grave to Cradle to Now

A father's first hand account

The Health Care Professional Edition

Using the collaterally damaged family as a lifesaving and healing instrument and other observations by the father of a traumatically brain injured son

For Doctors, Nurses, Therapists, Educators, Patients, Families, Friends, Human Resources ...

Ian Powell

Marrette Publishing

www.marrette.cc/publishing.html

Some of the material in this book was first published, in different form, in *Navigating the System of Brain Injury - A Resource Manual For Individuals and Families Impacted by Brain Injury*

Permission to use that material is gratefully acknowledged.

Library and Archives Canada Cataloguing in Publication

Powell, Ian, 1944

From Grave to Cradle to Now - The Health Care Professional Edition / Ian Powell.

ISBN 978-0-9880073-0-7 soft
ISBN 978-0-09880073-1-4 e-Book
ISBN 978-0-9880073-2-1 hard cover

1. Surviving traumatic brain injury—Patients—Health professionals—Families—Memoir. 2. Acquired and traumatic brain injuries in families—Patients—Family relationships—Canada. 3. Parents, families and friends of patients with brain injuries—Canada—Memoir. 4. Text—Nurses—Doctors—Psychologists—Sociologists. 5. Subjects—Coma care—Critical care—Using family as instruments—Entrainment—Blood Harmony—Nursing arts—Care giving I. Title.

Design by Jon McCallum

Printed in the United States of America

10 9 8 7 6 5 4 3 2 1

Contents

Preface

Three individuals drew this story from me, from bed to book as it were, in successive stages.

Chris Foot asked me to speak to the *Men's Breakfast* of the local *United Church*.

This group invites members, authors and other guest speakers on a wide range of subjects including Western abuse of Africa; logic; the evolution of door-to-door milk delivery; a celebrated locally-born international artist; pilots on flying; political campaigning; high tech entrepreneurship; and German history and the machinations of East Germany. Talks are given by members and outside experts. The speakers are invited in order to stimulate thought and community.

Preparing that talk forced me to understand, organize and condense events into a 40-minute presentation.

Most attendees knew me; a couple knew Drew, my son and this story's central figure. As much public speaking as I have done, it was a minor miracle that I was able to give the talk only 7-months after Drew's accident. That was particularly true as, unexpectedly, I saw the audience barely withholding tears at times. Fortunately, we were also able to let off pressure by laughing in the appropriate places.

Two years later, Ramona Bray, Drew's psychotherapist and a clinical social worker, asked Drew to write an account and asked me to write a father's first person account of my journey with

Drew. She felt that our 3-year-long stories would be helpful additions to the next issue of her *Navigating the System of Brain Injury - A Resource Manual For Individuals and Families Impacted by Brain Injury*. Every two years, she publishes the guide for families, patients, health care and other professionals. Apparently such male, father, or father-son accounts are very rare.

I hesitated some months before starting the project but, not only did the process prove to be cathartic, it benefited our family's ongoing journey. Ramona provided insightful questions for me to address. These questions, coupled with knowing the intended readership, brought focus and discipline to my writing. The earlier 40-minute talk became 30 pages, as writing unearthed suppressed memories and revealed insights.

Reading that text some 4 months later, a modest, un-nameable mentor to budding Florence Nightingales, a retired faculty member who taught nursing students for two-plus decades, suggested that if I added certain content the text would be a very useful resource for nursing educators. As I had no professional expertise, I agreed only if she would guide me. Several months later she sent that enhanced draft to several institutions: a hospital and a nursing school. The last two expressed purchase interest. For me, that acceptance legitimized the value of the content.

Thereby emboldened, I sought more validation and critiques by contacting a range of relevant professionals, institutions and associations in North America and other English speaking countries. The responses have been universally positive— encouraging.

This step by step process encouraged me to stick with **my** voice in writing the first person account rather than the drier, technical, business-speak that I am usually called on to write. This approach encouraged me to keep it conversational which may balance the didactic flowing from observations, reflection and lessons learned. I hope that combination works for you.

Acknowledgement

My greatest thanks, by far, go to Drew. Our son has always brought immense richness to my life. He inspires. He embraces this chapter in his life with insight, dedication, and self-discipline. I'm certain that you will draw a similar conclusion after reading the *Drew Writes* chapter which he contributed to Ramona's *Reference Guide* and which is based on remarks he made to a 2010 conference of health care professionals.

I give particular thanks to my wife, Drew's mother Rachel, who has and continues to be strongly central to our caregiving team. I provide examples throughout the book.

We all know that we were fortunate to have such a strong core and extended family. Their mutual love and support, with maturity, intelligence and compassion, enabled all of us to survive this journey stronger and healthier than when we entered it. They included Drew's brothers Neil, JJ and his girlfriend Alexandra, and Drew's Aunt Marie and Uncle Christian all of whom suffered the bomb blast with us. Neil's Angella joined our core team not long after. Several agreed to read this account and made helpful contributions

Drew's friends and colleagues are a class unto themselves. They suffered. Several were active daily in practical ways and in ways that emotionally connected us in a direct and positive way to the vast community that Drew had touched. They revealed to us the high regard in which Drew is held. Their love, prayers and active support for Drew, for us and for each other have been truly inspiring. This widely diverse group of people displayed a high level of mutual support, of community in the old-fashioned sense that is wonderful and very encouraging to see.

We must thank the many friends, neighbours and colleagues who supported us then and now. I provide a few examples in the book.

I estimate that 180 health care professionals saved, cared for and still participate in rehabilitating Drew. I don't know and can't name all of them. We have been able to thank some of them directly, and, on behalf of Drew's family, friends and colleagues I now thank them collectively. Most were in St. Michael's Hospital, the others were in St. Joseph's and Bridgepoint Rehabilitation. Several times during his recovery and additional surgeries when Drew and his mother Rachel and I would enter NeuroTrauma ICU or run into the staff in the hospital we would thank them. They said that they seldom get to see the healthy, recovered patient. They were all grateful and obviously pleased to meet the normal Drew who was a far cry from the battered Drew they had saved and cared for.

With their permission, I thank two doctors who were extremely important to Drew's survival and recovery. Both were part of the initial emergency team. Both conducted at least two subsequent surgeries and related consultations. Dr. Richard Perrin is Drew's neurosurgeon and Dr. James Mahoney is his plastic surgeon. Rachel and I have been privileged to be present when they consulted with Drew and to see their obvious professional expertise and the warmth they bring to their discussions with Drew and with us, both pre- and post-surgery. Both have downplayed their expertise, Dr. Perrin even going so far to say that he is "just a technician." We know better.

Other professionals important to Drew and to us include physiatrists, ophthalmologic surgeons, rehabilitation specialists and the doctors in NeuroTrauma ICU, one of whom, Dr. Andrew Baker, I mention in the body of the book.

We also thanked the seven police officers who had recovered Drew and turned him over to the EMS ambulance. The sergeant was shocked to learn the severity of Drew's injuries and to hear that he had spent 111 days in hospital.

Drew's ongoing recovery also owes a lot to his employing company's compassion and active support, from the President, Human Resources, his immediate bosses and colleagues.

Drew's ongoing security in a financial sense was aided substantially by a wonderful firm of lawyers—Theall Group LLP. I can't recommend them highly enough for their professionalism, bull-dog determination and compassion.

I am grateful for the many that were necessary for the very existence of this book. Chris Foot, the Chairman of the Men's Breakfast, set the ball rolling.

Particular thanks goes to Ramona R. Bray (CYW, MSW, RSW, OSP, Certified Clinical Psychotherapist Specialization In Trauma Rehabilitation) not only for calling the initial text into being but most of all for her ongoing tremendous help to all of us, particularly to Drew, guiding us along our unmapped journey to each new normal, whatever that is to be. The Bridgepoint Rehabilitation Hospital gave us her name and a glowing referral.

The final stage in the creation of the book is due to the unnameable retired faculty member and educator of nurses who saw a specific potential for a professionally focused version. I valued her suggestion, in part, because for decades she educated health care students with respect to sociology, psychology (health, social, developmental), conflict resolution, and organizational behaviour as it pertained to their jobs. She had the important insight and expertise that I needed. I am indebted to her for much discussion, insight, ideas and counsel over six months.

I am very grateful to the four impressive individuals endorsing the book who, from their diverse health care experience, showed me that the book would also have value beyond the acquired and the traumatic brain injury communities (ABI/TBI).

Another modest woman provided invaluable editing assistance, helping me to clarify and thereby to discover, and forcing me to justify why I should break a few rules. Coincidentally, years ago she tutored Drew; now he tutors us.

I am very pleased that Drew's brother, JJ, did the design and layout for this book.

Introduction to the Health Care Professional Edition

Apparently not many fathers, men, write first person trauma accounts.

In my childhood, my Aunt freed our songless, grumpy budgie from the jaws of her cat. It was shaken up badly and bleeding slightly. Moments later, it started singing, which it did until it died years later. That tale came to mind when I realized that, in the past two years, I have become more talkative, processing our current journey with my critically injured son to anyone who would listen. Attacks of the budgies appear out of the blue, like Tourettes, kind of alarming and charming. When I realized that was happening as I walked the neighbourhood, I began to take therapy-dog with me to protect my reputation. I'm better now, thanks.

Health care professionals (HCPs) first asked me to write about my experience for the benefit of other collaterally damaged families of the traumatically injured. Then other HCPs asked me to augment that material specifically for the benefit of health care professionals, even though I am not a health care expert. Presumably the request was because I have other expertise including multi-year, daily experience with a traumatically injured patient and months and years of experience up-close-and-personal with health care professionals and the hospital system.

These experts believe that it would be helpful for you to read about and to visualize the lives of patients and their families, as those lives evolve together when you are not present. Also, the experts thought you would benefit from seeing your profession and the health care system through the eyes of those participating from the other side of the bed. To this task I bring observational and formal experience as entrepreneur, executive and management consultant, and a limited amount of expertise gained as volunteer, advisor and consultant to the head of a cancer research foundation and clinic. This text has been reviewed, edited and augmented by health care professionals, some of whom are identified in the Preface.

The initial third is the heart of the book. It quotes verbatim the raw, selected, daily Facebook and Journal entries that recorded the initial bomb blast to our lives followed by the evolution of the gravely uncertain present. I have augmented these entries with previously undisclosed facts, observations and analysis. The next two thirds contain separate observations for the specific use of health care professionals, on the one hand, and other collaterally damaged families, on the other.

Understandably, to enhance patient outcomes health care professionals and the collaterally damaged families need to work together; but, apparently, don't always do so. It is as if we speak different languages, inhabit different worlds—and we do. I hope that this text will provide insights that will enable you to lead rag-tag teams of collaterally damaged; turning them into effective caregiver teams. By doing so, you will simultaneously heal them and enable them to pull their loved ones into viable new normals.

This text also delves into experiences that are very hard to accept, difficult to describe and almost impossible to explain. As a result, I hope that during your formal education and health care practice you keep a mind open to unorthodox insights yielding increased professional effectiveness and satisfaction.

As horrific as our journey was in the beginning, our family members have benefited in ways that the general public, the recently brain-injured family and perhaps even some health care professionals will have difficulty comprehending. Our shared experience has brought us great personal growth, greater respect for each other, stronger selves and relationships, greater appreciation for the things of life of true value, enabled insight, and, as strange as it may seem, yielded much humour.

Apparently, those benefits were evolving early on. In the maelstrom, we could not recognize them but professionals could. Drew's young GP came to visit the comatose Drew in NeuroTrauma ICU. She could do nothing for Drew but she stayed more than half an hour to talk with my wife and me. As she left she said, "I don't know how you have been able to cope so well."

Writing this text was very hard at times but ultimately both illuminating and cathartic. As I write and speak to interested groups and process lessons for business groups, I continue to learn about all the normals we have lived and are living. As a health care professional you will see things in this material that I haven't yet perceived and may never grasp.

I hope that you will see, as I have been told, that our story has universality and applicability beyond parent/child, male/male and brain injury relationships.

I hope that you don't mind, but I have used pseudonyms for close family in order to write more openly about our experience. Also, you will notice that my tenses are a mixture of present and past. I started to make corrections but stopped when I realized this is an accurate reflection of how I relate to those events today. Those events are still in my present. I don't *remember* them so much as I *relive* them. No doubt you will note my warped relationship with time.

To conclude our story, for the moment, Drew provides his observations and insights which he wrote to help other brain injured patients.

Ian Powell
February 2012
Toronto

FROM GRAVE TO CRADLE TO NOW

Grave

That first Saturday in April promised to be the first beautiful day of spring. We were expecting our eldest son, 32-year-old Drew, to arrive for the weekend from his loft in the west end of Toronto. From age 11 he had lived where we still live but from his first year at Ryerson University, he lived in Toronto. As a 20-year-old wouldn't you?

We were looking forward to seeing him, on his own for a few days—a rare occurrence.

For six years he had been working at a high pressure job providing the top level support for corporations around the world. His company is a major player in the World Wide Web. In the coming week, Drew was to start the new job that the company had created so that they could take better advantage of his relationship success with clients.

As much as he loved his work, he loved more being a composer and performer of electronic music. While still in his teens, he had earned a global reputation for his ground-breaking Internet performances for which he had been written up internationally in *Music and Computers Magazine* and in the *Internet Handbook*.

As I was driving about doing errands, suddenly I had a feeling of apprehension: an irrational awareness of a train and a strong impulse to phone Drew. I suppressed the impulse, rationalizing that calling at 10:15 on a Saturday morning would probably wake him.

0 : H   12:10 PM – The Call

At 12:10, vacuuming the kitchen, I didn't hear the phone. Minutes later, my wife Rachel, handed me the phone saying gravely, "Listen to this. It's the police about Drew. I'm going to get ready to leave."

The recording stated that the police had found Drew near tracks in West Toronto bleeding from a serious head injury.

I phoned the sergeant at the scene who gave me the basic information including that Drew was OK but had a fractured skull and lost a lot of blood from a head wound. Drew had given the police his name and spelled it out, but wasn't answering any other questions. He had walked with the police some 300 metres to the vehicles. The officer said that they didn't know exactly what had happened, as there were no witnesses, but they assumed that he had been hit by a train. Apparently, someone in an apartment about a block away had called 911 to report seeing somebody staggering along the tracks. The police had then stopped all trains in West Toronto.

"A train!? He's seriously injured but he survived the accident. He talked and walked so he will be fine," we thought.

I told the sergeant that we would meet him in 45 minutes at Saint Joseph's Health Centre just off the Queensway. He advised me to drive carefully and not to speed.

En route, we called Neil and JJ our two other sons. The police had already called Neil. He was on his way to the hospital; so was youngest brother JJ, with his girlfriend Alexandra. Rachel's sister Marie and brother-in-law Christian were on their way as well.

1 : H   1:00 PM – Hospital Number 1 – St. Joseph's

On arrival, by accident Rachel and I walked into the off-limits Emergency Triage Room. We saw Drew's unmistakable legs and, walking closer, saw with great relief that he had no apparent injuries below his nose. From there on up, his head was wrapped.

The waiting room for the seven of us was a claustrophobic 8x15 feet. I went to meet with the police.

Minutes later the Emergency Room (ER) doctor told us that their X-rays and computed tomography (CT) scan showed that Drew's brain injuries were so serious that they were sending him by special ambulance either to Sunnybrook or St. Michael's hospitals, whichever could treat him quickest. This was more serious than we thought, but Drew had talked to the police and walked with them to the ambulance. We had no doubt that he would be fine.

2 : H 2:40 PM – Ambulance

The ambulance crew invited Rachel and me to accompany Drew in the ambulance. She sat with Drew; I sat with the driver. A parking lot pot-hole caused several metallic crashing noises in back but the EMS technician replied that all was fine. As he slowly drove onto the street, the driver called dispatch asking them to tell St. Michael's ER that we would be there in 9 minutes. "Good luck," I thought to myself. "It's mid-afternoon on the first nice Saturday of spring, so the 8 kilometers of streets between us in West Toronto and St. Mike's in Central Toronto would be jammed with cars and pedestrians. Either you're fibbing, to make certain that the emergency team is ready when we arrive, or you know some route that I don't."

We turned east onto Queen Street West. As we drove through the first main intersection, the driver pulled into the left lane, accelerating head-on into the oncoming traffic. Then he turned on every siren and flashing light the ambulance had. Suddenly, I felt enormous fear. "What does the driver know that I don't?"

We drove very quickly either on the wrong side of the street or in the centre of the street on a frequently weaving lane that the ambulance driver created with the forced cooperation of the traffic. We passed Trinity Bellwood Park, restaurants, and stores, places Drew and I had visited together, as well as his ex-girlfriend's condo. I wondered, "Is this the last time Drew will ever be here?"

In spite of two initially-uncooperative motorists, we arrived at St. Michael's in less than 9 minutes.

My earlier lack of fear had not been the result of denial, but rather the result of the positive police report about Drew's behaviour after the injury, my own observation of Drew, the calm professionalism of the medical staff, but most of all, my ignorance.

3 : H 3:00 PM – Hospital Number 2 – St. Michael's

In the St. Michael's ER, a waiting team of 20 emergency staff descended on Drew for half an hour. The ambulance crew took us into an adjacent waiting room and brought us coffee. Then they briefed us on the next steps including that the emergency team estimated that the surgery would take 1-2 hours. A nurse sent us to the 9th floor NeuroTrauma ICU Waiting Room for the duration. Briefly in denial I thought, "We don't belong here with these exhausted, grim-faced people." I'm sure that they thought the same about us.

At 9:30, more than 4 ½ hours since the start of surgery, an assisting surgeon appeared.

9 : H 9:30 PM – Assisting Surgeon's Description of Drew's Situation

I stopped the surgeon from starting his report until we could collect all seven of us into the empty waiting room. We were all standing. As the surgeon made small talk, I noticed that the pant legs of his hospital greens were soaked in Drew's blood.

His five-minute briefing was detailed and matter-of-fact. Drew had:

- Lost a lot of blood and had received quite a few transfusions
- A fractured vertebrae in his neck

- Two broken ribs, bleeding in the chest and a partially collapsed lung
- Badly swollen eyes and possible irreparable damage to the eyes
- Chipped teeth, a broken nose and badly-fractured eye sockets, forehead and left side of his skull
- Bone fragments in his brain which they had removed. His brain was bleeding at the frontal lobe, the left temporal lobe and at the base of the brain where it joins the brain stem at the spine
- An extremely badly swelling brain that the doctors can do nothing about except to let it swell by removing the front half of his skull, from his eyebrows and ears to the top of his head
- Drew was in the deepest coma short of a vegetative state.

Sensing the devastation that his information had created, from compassion, but without apparent conviction, the surgeon added, "Of course he's young. He could beat the odds and survive."

We plunge into numbing depths, our lived *normal* ripped from us forever. Initially, we are all so stunned that we can't console each other. One brother faints to the floor. One brother (a former ocean lifeguard, trained and experienced in dealing with traumatic injuries) is distraught. Alexandra, his wonderful girlfriend of a year who barely knows Drew, is equally devastated and appears lost. With "JJ needs you," I send her to console my son.

10:H 9: 45 PM - The Quiet Room & Shifts

Hospital staff take us to the Quiet Room dedicated to such circumstances. It has a pull-out bed we don't discover for three days, laying on the floor instead. We displace a family originally from Mauritius, the young wife and mother of which was hit two days before by a young drunk driver. We bond through grief. Two days later, they take her off life support.

11:H

10:45 PM - Sitting with Drew

An hour later, after staff settle Drew into the NeuroTrauma ICU, my wife and I start one hour round-the-clock shifts by his side.

As I pass the nurse busily dedicated to Drew 24/7 and enter his side-curtained ICU cubicle, I see a lifeless Drew lying in subdued lighting, connected by at least a dozen tubes and wires to about 24 square feet of instrumentation rising behind him, quietly beeping or making other gentle noises. Drew's wrapped, swelling head has already more than doubled in size.

I sit, take his hand in mine and kiss it. "Hi Drew; its Dad. I love you Drew."

Then in the blink of an eye, I had this internal conversation. "How do I survive this?... You have to accept that Drew is dead.... Given his extensive brain damage, if he survives he might never be able to hear, see, talk, or feed himself. Perhaps dying is best.... No, I will accept him, whatever his condition.... Now what do I have to do to bring him back?"

In the blink of an eye.

At that moment, an electric shock passed from his hand to mine, similar to strong static electricity, but not unpleasant. "He's in there!" I thought.

But it was much more than that. Now I realise that that electric shock was calling me to experience Drew beyond his battered body, to experience a healthy Drew who was very present to me; and I to him. We had communicated; connection in its purest form. I recall that this essence of Drew was healthy, calm and vibrant, quite different from and independent of the battered body. Reliving his presence, I wonder now if he may also have been observing, evaluating, deciding or even re-deciding. Then I experienced a deep, lasting peace. And so it has been.

Part of Rachel's own bedside dialogue was: "Whatever God decides I will accept."

And so, we passed the night.

With that peace also came awareness that all my fears were not gone but were simply stored in a Sack of Dread that I now carried on my back and feared would rupture. Also came a partial defence against rupture, withdrawing into a rolling 10 seconds of existence, the eternal present in which we live for many months.

The past and the future were banished; as was any part of the world more than 10 seconds away. For this reason, for months we kept radios and TV off and stopped reading newspapers.

Why is my internal dialogue important? I think that I had to experience Drew's death to ensure his resurrection. That sentence may appear to border on the sacrilegious; I don't mean it to. Perhaps there are useful resonances there for others to consider. I cannot—not yet.

Had I attempted to save Drew from death, instead of striving to bring Drew2 to life, would I have become so emotionally destroyed that I could not have helped him? Would I have been so focused on myself that I would not have had enough energy, will or mental resources to help him? Would my fear and emotions have drained me to the point of impotence?

Upon reflection, there might be a debate about what could be characterized as the obligation to the injured versus an overriding obligation to the self—in order that you survive so that you can help the injured. However, is there not always obligation to our injured child NEVER to give up, to fight by every means possible to prevent them dying? Was I selfish in accepting that Drew was dead? Or was it absolutely necessary in order that he might transcend death, that his vital essence be reunited with a viable body?

It was three years after the event, while writing this book, that I became aware of this alternative. However, I cannot consider or discuss it further for to do so would require me to go within myself to a place and time I can never truly visit again because of the Sack of Dread.

GRAVE

Chronology: Facebook and Journal

The following are reduced and annotated, selected items from our Facebook postings or, where indicated, from my journal. I have kept the grammar and spelling of the Facebook postings. The elapsed time is indicated in the margin by **H**our, **D**ay, **M**onth and **Y**ear.

24:H

Facebook Posting # 1 - Coma
Sunday, April 6 - morning

Dear friends of Drew,

Drew was in a serious accident on the morning of Saturday, April 5. He was admitted in to the hospital with severe head trauma, and underwent extensive surgery. He is in critical condition and is now being stabilized. We are told that from now until Tuesday evening is a critical period for him.

His friends and community have always been supportive, and I know that he would like to see your wishes once he gets through this. So post on the wall, send messages, spread the word.

It's a tough time for all of us, and him most of all. We know he'll appreciate your prayers.

Please pass this information and group on to anyone who knows him.

We'll be posting updates when we have any more information.

—Drew's Family

Note: With daylight came renewed resolve to get busy, to bring Drew back, or rather, to bring Drew2 to life.

Drew had survived 12 of the first 36 critical hours. His head appeared to have swollen to nearly three times its normal size. That observation no longer shocks us.

The morning of the second day, exhausted, stressed and full of adrenalin toxins is when you begin to plan as best you can. Later still, on the third day, you confirm the evolving dotted lines of responsibility. However, you have to remain flexible because of the patient's unresolved status, and because when exhaustion and stress knock everyone off their game, others have to step in.

There are extraordinary tasks that the family must address once the patient is settled into NeuroTrauma ICU: bedside schedules, deciding and advocating on behalf of the patient, logistics (food, accommodation, travel, children, parents, and pets), notification and communications (relatives, friends, employers).

We agreed upon, and settled immediately into, our respective roles. Rachel became the primary, within arms-length caregiver spending most time with Drew and dealing with ICU staff. Neil and JJ took on the role of connecting Drew with the outside world: Facebook and Drew's friends. I straddled both areas. I spent lots of time with Drew and dealt with logistics, hospital administration, Drew's employer, the police, lawyers, selected friends and colleagues of Drew.

I became aware that our relatives and friends were now our greatest risk to puncture our Sacks of Dread. They represented the past and the future. They would be emotional and they would be needy. Each would ask the same questions we dare not contemplate, specifically "What happened?" and "How is Drew?"

On his own initiative Sunday morning, almost exactly 24 hours after Drew was injured, brother Neil created the Facebook site "Drew Powell is in the hospital…" It provides these selected postings.

In April 2008, I knew little about Facebook. However, when Neil arrived at the hospital and told me what he had done, I knew that he had a created a very important tool and so it proved to be for many reasons. The first posting was Day 2 at 10:20 a.m. Ultimately 800 people registered; there were 47 pages of daily updates, 948 messages and 66 pictures posted by others. This site fed thousands of people via other web sites run by both Drew's industry and music communities. They often carried our postings and hyperlinked to our site.

Registrations and postings grew rapidly and the latter were agonizing. Barely two hours from the time that he created the Facebook site, Neil brought in the first messages which we read and re-read to Drew. The nurses gathered around to listen. One nurse said, "He must be a wonderful person for so many people to love him so much." I noticed that Drew was becoming a person to them, more than a patient for whom dying was now just a formality.

That Sunday afternoon, we discussed Facebook and how to use it. In the first two hours over 100 people registered to receive updates. It made us aware that we were at the centre of an information vacuum.

We knew that:

- We needed to prepare people—at the various stages, whatever they might be

- Information needed to be edited, authentic and reliable and we needed to head off the inevitable rumours and

- Readers needed to be able to move from being distraught to DOING something useful—for their sake as well as for Drew's.

29

We knew we would benefit immediately from the Facebook site by eliminating all incoming phone calls and by not having to deal with non-essential people who would eat up time and energy and would risk rupturing the Sack of Dread. Also, while Neil or I did the daily postings, this daily informal collective process saved all of us energy by updating a shared message, helped us recognize that day's critical elements and helped us focus on the positive. It was information push; condensed, efficient and safe. Moreover, the process effectively united us as a mutually supporting team rather than individuals operating independently and therefore risking chaos and acting at cross-purposes.

Sunday morning, being on message got a trial run at the hospital where, coincidentally, L'Arche had a core member on the same floor. At the elevator we bump into senior L'Arche assistants who are very close to us and who are also health care professionals.

There were 3 groups that were low risk to puncture our Sacks of Dread: hospital staff, families of the at-risk patients in the other 36 NeuroTrauma ICU beds and our friends from the local L'Arche communities for intellectually handicapped adults. Rachel was on their Board of Directors and we had enjoyed 20-year friendships with numerous assistants and core members. Through L'Arche, we knew many people with serious intellectual and physical handicaps and their caregivers. We could relate with these friends and they with us at a level that did not need words. The senior hospital social worker also turned out to have once been an assistant at L'Arche.

Monday morning an Anglican Priest, a close friend from L'Arche, dressed in official purple and crosses arrived at ICU looking like a bishop, to prevent being denied access to Drew.

To my great surprise the president of Drew's company called me and asked what he could do. This was a welcome call from outside our rolling 10 second reality.

24:H Minor update
Sunday, April 6 - night

I've been getting a lot of requests about where to send flowers and cards. Drew's in the Intensive Care Unit, and from what I understand, probably will be for another ten days. ICU seems to be like a lock-down, and there really isn't any place for teddy bears or flowers. My family also has no permanent place in the hospital, so there's nowhere for anything to be put.

Visitation is limited, and at the moment, only family members are allowed. But you can send your wishes in other ways. I've been printing out all your wonderful messages, and have given them to my mother to read to Drew. Drew is in a coma, but I know in my heart that he can hear us—so please keep those messages coming!

I know the information is sparse at this point, but we're all just trying to hold it together. We'll fill you in as we know more.

Lots of love to you all,

—Neil

47:H Movement?
Monday, April 7 - early morning

The staff at the ICU are regularly testing Drew's awareness. Drew is apparently reacting to some stimulus, although I'm told that at this point it's all involuntary. Nonetheless, this is a *good* sign, as I understand it. Keep the prayers coming.

My dad wanted me to share with all of you that my family is reading all the postings that you're putting up, and we're grateful for the loving response of so many people and for the offers of help.

—Neil

Note: On Monday the shock to Drew's colleagues virtually shut down the office. Monday night, coinciding with the end of the

31

critical 36 hours, a group of Drew's secular friends held a prayer vigil for Drew in a local park. Soon there would be Muslim prayer vigils for him in a Mosque in Dubai, and similar ceremonies held by Buddhists in Toronto, a convent of nuns in Haiti, and churches in Canada, England and Australia.

Prayers were needed. Compounding our distress was the fact that at the first hospital the police had told me that they were investigating Drew's injury as the consequence of a possible attempted suicide.

Why have I not mentioned this before? Because our focus on returning Drew to life was so all-consuming that it pushed the improbable suicide possibility completely to the back of our minds.

That would change and we would address it over time in a variety of ways. I was aware that the medical staff had this information and the police had questioned his roommates so the theory was out there, feeding people's quite natural desire to know. Had and would this theory negatively affect Drew's treatment by hospital staff?

The facts did not appear to support a self-harm theory but it could not be ignored. First, I decided that we would never mention it on Facebook. Second, I realized that there were individuals who would be agonizing to a far greater extent than the rest of his friends. Therefore, during the first week, I made a point of meeting with his loft-mates and Neil and I met with one of Drew's close friends. From my own experience I knew that any guilt that they felt could be quite irrational. I felt that it would be important for them that Drew's family give them the *facts* directly; absolve them of any responsibility that they felt—as best as we could; and, let them know that Drew's family did not hold them responsible. It was also important to give them the chance to talk. I offered to find them counselling, as I did to all of Drew's friends, if they needed professional help to deal with their grief.

In an interesting way, absolving them helped me to process my own guilt. Each family member had to deal with their respective anger with Drew and their sense of guilt for what we may have not seen, said or not said, done or not done. My wife and I never attempted to discuss it. I discussed it with the boys, one on one. After several weeks, we met as a group with the hospital psychologist who specialized in suicide. Surprisingly, she said that in her years of experience she had never met with an entire family.

This session proved to be very helpful to us in many ways. The timing was perfect. She grounded us, getting us away from the fearful by explaining the reality. She also provided us with concrete steps to take going forward. She provided us with a methodology for dealing with Drew if and when he healed enough that either he remembered what happened or asked why he was injured. She also suggested that he would need counselling either to deal with any recollection, to help him understand, or to prevent a reoccurrence. The key point was, "Let Drew come to you." Also, she provided us with an opportunity to ask the questions that we dared not ask each other.

Later, multiple sets of psychiatrists determined that Drew presented no evidence either of past or present intent to self-harm. Drew had no memory of how he was injured or the lead up to it. He was extremely shocked at the self-harm question. However, accepting that it might be the case, he expressed forcefully the determination to make certain that he would never allow himself to get into such a state of mind.

The kicker, what we did not know for nearly a year, was that the police had closed their file that first day with the comment, "It is unknown exactly how the victim received his injuries." They had no eyewitnesses and were missing answers to who, how, where, when, what and why. Drew was found mid-morning staggering near tracks and bridges a kilometre down the tracks from where he lived. The tracks were only 60 metres from his loft through a large hole in a fence. While the police's main guess was that a train hit him, the nature of his serious injuries, limited to from his cheekbones up, was inconsistent with the theory that a 150-pound man had been hit by a moving 150-ton engine. We had been asking ourselves that very question for most of that year.

74:H Full-to-brimming with love, reading, boom box
Tuesday, April 8 - noon

My family and I are really astounded—but of course not surprised—by the outpouring in this Facebook group and from elsewhere. Over 100 people joined since I looked at it yesterday at noon, and ten more have joined in the five minutes I've been sitting here. Drew is truly loved, and it shows. He touched many people in his life, and he has many more yet to.

I am really amazed by the healing circle, and I want to thank Lisa for organizing that. I wish I had heard in time to be able to come; our phones are off in the hospital, and I don't have my computer there.

Last night, I sat down for a half hour and read as many of your wall postings to Drew as I could. I know that my father also read many of them earlier that day. We're reading and re-reading them.

We're arranging to set up a little boom box to play his music and DJ mixes to him (sorry, no subwoofers in ICU). I'd like to arrange for all of you to record audio messages to him. I'm a little frazzled right now, and was hoping someone could spearhead the logistics of this. Can someone take this on? It would be great if there was a simple way that even Luddites could record a message to him. Please let me know if this gets going.

My mother left the hospital for the first time last night to get some sleep. She's been by him since he was first admitted. He's really truly blessed to have her—we all are.

Drew's condition is still critical but stable, and there hasn't been much change since yesterday, which we're told is good news. He's still in a coma, but regularly reacting to stimulus. It all kind of freaks me out, but I take comfort in what the nurses are telling us.

I know that people have been passing my e-mail address on in case others have no Facebook account. That's wonderful—please keep that going. Being Communications Director for this has proved to be incredibly time-consuming, and I can't guarantee that I'll be able to respond to all the e-mails, but if they're addressed to Drew I promise I'll print them out for him.

Keep up the good energy. It's getting through to him, I know it.

Much love to all of you and your loved ones,

—Neil

Note: Neil arranged for us to have an early meeting this morning near the hospital in the offices of a lawyer he knew who specialized in insurance litigation. Neil correctly sensed that we might need to do something but there was no way we could yet be proactive other than be mindful of potential problems if Drew survived. The lawyer gave us a sense of statutory limitations and realities. Later, when Drew's company's disability insurance firm became a problem, this lawyer helped me conduct a "beauty contest" of potential law firms. I chose one of the lawyers he recommended and, to our collective surprise, we won within a week of sending to the insurance company our first collectively and carefully crafted letter.

94:H Rachel and I return home, briefly, for the first time
Wednesday, April 9 · morning · Journal

Mid-morning day four we returned home for the first time in order to change clothes, pick up more changes of clothes since Rachel was going to stay with her sister, Marie, who lived much closer to the hospital and was attending every day.

To reinforce with the medical staff the awareness of the vital, beloved Drew, to hang by his ICU bed I picked up, not a portrait of Drew, but a large candid family photo with a very lively Drew in it.

Just before we left, we saw the beautiful arrangement of flowers that Drew sent to Rachel on her birthday, the day before he was injured. I left Rachel photographing the bouquet from many different angles; the complex symbolism was too much for me. Waiting outside for Rachel so we could return to the hospital, I started despondently tidying up the front yard. The sound of nearby screeching brakes made me look up. An SUV was stopped, straddling the middle of the street and a woman was getting out from behind the wheel. She was a good, forthright friend and neighbour striding towards me with a tremendous look of care and concern and shock on her face. Her sudden appearance finally ripped open the Sack of Dread. I was losing it big time and had to clench my jaw exceptionally tight to stay in control. Of course, that made me look even worse which shocked her into mouth-open silence. I fought hard to control myself as I didn't know if a meltdown then and there would incapacitate me at a time when I was needed. Later she said that I had looked so absolutely awful that it had put her in shock, preventing her from melting down, fortunately. I don't know how we drove safely back to the hospital.

102:H

Thumbs up!
Wednesday, April 9 - afternoon

Holy crap. According to the nurses, this morning, Drew gave a squeeze and a thumbs up on command. Holy crap!

Drew is apparently no longer in a regular coma (whatever "regular" is), but during this brief bout of consciousness he was struggling against the respirator and working himself up into a tizzy, and tizzies are bad for him at this stage. The staff sedated him and he's now in an induced coma to allow him to rest and heal. I think he is in a lot of pain. I can only imagine what it must feel like to be inside his head right now.

Thank you very much to those who dropped CDs off. It turns out that he now needs low stimulation, but you can bet I'll be playing those CDs when he's ready for it.

Thumbs up!

—Neil

Note: Drew's youngest brother, JJ, had a most difficult time. He was completing his two years of graduate animation training at Sheridan College, one of the top animation schools in the world. Within the next three weeks, he had to complete animations for his portfolio both in order to pass his course and to have a portfolio of his work to show industry employers including the likes of Disney, Industrial Light and Magic and game companies. They came to Sheridan's Industry Day in early May each year to evaluate and hire animators.

While JJ wanted to be with Drew we told him that Drew would want him to complete his course. The rest of us were able to handle all of Drew's needs. If JJ were to be needed, he was only 45 minutes away.

Still devastated, he went back to Sheridan. His distress was compounded by the fact that six years before a train killed a high school friend, which had devastated him and their close circle of friends. It must have been a huge challenge for JJ to find the willpower, energy and self-discipline to NOT focus on Drew 24 hours of the day. His girlfriend Alexandra, who worked nearby as a consulting engineer, provided invaluable support to him and saw to it that he got through the next month successfully—he was hired by an animation company. Knowing that he was in her loving and capable hands took an enormous load off us so that we could focus on Drew. Alexandra and JJ marry three years later.

11:D Infection
Thursday, April 10 - late afternoon

Drew's developed an infection in one of his lungs and is now being dosed with antibiotics. You smokers out there, take note: the nurses tell me that smokers are more likely to develop infections in their lungs in critical care, and infections are serious problems in this state.

So, why don't some of you target your prayers to his lungs, and the rest of you keep focussing on his head? Let's make sure all of him is covered.

We seem to have amassed a large group of people who are all directing positive energy towards Drew, and it's a very lovely thing.

I also realize that there are many others out there also in need of positive energy, and I think Drew would love to be able to make use of this situation to help others. I can't ask him, of course, but he's an upstanding chap and I'll just assume on his behalf.

If anyone out there has someone in need of prayers and good energy, please post about them on the discussion thread that I've started so we can all send some good vibes their way. All of you sending positive energy out, please add these people to your prayers.

—Neil

11:D Drew's progress – Neil is exhausted & has the flu; tapping out a beat
Wednesday, April 16

Drew's brother, Neil, has created this site and has been posting updates, among many other ways that he has supported his brother over the past 12 days. However, he is wiped at the moment so he has entrusted me with administrator status so that I can post updates.

Drew is more aware, responding to questions by nodding, thumbs up, wiggling his toes, and making a fist. I noticed that he seemed to be tapping out different beat sequences with the fingers of his right hand, first on the bed and then on my hand. I replied to each sequence by tapping his hand, repeating his sequence. What's the music that he is channeling?

Keep up your wonderful, powerful focus on reducing the swelling of Drew's brain. We want to hear that music.

The diversity of powers concentrated on healing Drew inspire awe. That Drew could touch so many people so profoundly, in his life before and in his need now, is remarkable. It is a tribute to Drew and a tribute to you - it is a lesson in the power of "one".

Ian - Drew's father

13:D Post surgery update #2
Rachel "joins" medical team
Friday, April 18 - evening

Today was a day of recovery for Drew. He was aware but sedated, only up to holding hands. The hospital staff wrestled successfully with his pain, low level lung infection, fluctuating temperature and high heart rate. it doesn't sound like a lot of activity but it was constant activity through the day. We received a thorough briefing from the senior plastic surgeon who operated on Drew yesterday.

If Drew's mother gets any closer to the medical staff they will start paying her. Child rearing provided an undergraduate course in medicine; this is our post-graduate course. …

The tentative plan for tomorrow is to remove the ventilator he has had inserted for the past two weeks. This will be a major improvement in Drew's quality of life. The fist that he made few days ago was in response to his mother's question to him about the level of irritation of the ventilator.

The removal of the ventilator does not mean automatically that he will be able to speak. Like each aspect of Drew's progress, the return of speech would be a gift.

We have had confirmation from other knowledgeable medical professionals that Drew's progress to date provides good indications.

Keep those prayers and vibes coming.

Ian

Note: I slept soundly. Before breakfast, I went to put clothes in the washing machine. On the way, I saw the hospital bag containing the black suede coat, shoes and clothes that Drew had been wearing when he was injured. All were heavily caked in blood. His shirt was scissored into tatters. His pants were missing. Perhaps the impulse to clean them was an instinctive, ritualistic means of affirming that he would live. Perhaps…

My whirling thoughts were nausea-making, forcing me to push away the Sack of Dread. What to do? If Drew were to survive, would he want them or not? If he were to die, would we want them or not? I was incapable of deciding. But I knew that I could not allow my family to see that blood. Almost on auto-pilot, I threw the blood soaked shoes into the washing machine and, except for the coat, put the rest of the clothes into the garbage which I took to the curb for pick-up that day.

On the way to the hospital I took Drew's coat to the dry cleaner. There, matter-of-factly I explained to the Korean immigrant owner that it was my son's coat and that the encrusted stain to be removed was blood. I said that there was no rush to get the coat back. He was stoic throughout. However since that day, the husband and wife owners always greet me with eye contact and a warm smile. When I bring in clothes for cleaning, from memory they write my name and phone number on the receipt. When I return to pick up clothes, often they bring my cleaned clothes to the counter even before I get there.

15:D First words "Drew Powell"
Sunday, April 20 - morning 8:00

"Drew Powell" were Drew's first words!

This morning the nurse asked him his name. When she asked him if he knew where he was, he replied, "Yup".

His voice is hoarse. He has now been off the ventilator for 24 hours.

I could hug you all! I may set off for the hospital in my pjs.

Ian

15:D "I love you." Leaf Buds, Rub, Ambient Music, Amazing/Miracle
Sunday, April 20 - evening 7:00

"I love you."

Drew spoke.

He slept for most of the day. But in the late afternoon he woke up somewhat. From time to time, usually when the nurse was helping him cough and clearing his breathing passages, he spoke a fair amount but for the most part it was not intelligible except for "More" and "Thank you." His voice is hoarse. For the most part it is low and of low energy. Frequently it is congested. The oxygen mask and the ambient sounds of the equipment mask it too.

But from time to time he spoke clearly. "The music calms me down," referred to the Ambient CD that Neil had prepared. "Rub" he said to his Aunt who had stopped rubbing the sole of his foot. And both his parents, separately, heard, "I love you."

On the day that the leaf buds opened on the trees outside the hospital Drew said, "I love you."

One of the nurses who admitted Drew to NeuroTrauma ICU 15 days ago was on duty today. Drew's mother, Rachel, said to her, "Drew said his name this morning. It is amazing." The nurse replied, "No, it is a miracle."

You all participate in that miracle. He still needs to get his heart rate down, clear the pneumonia and reduce further the swelling of his brain.

But as his recovery goes, this has been a remarkable day.

If his recovery continues at this rate, not so far off he should be able to tell you himself, "I love you."

And so do we.

Ian, Rachel, Drew, Neil and JJ

16:D Drew waves, sits up! Pretty good, all things considered Dr. doesn't expect him to be there.
Monday, April 21 — evening #2

Neil's report below is pretty remarkable. So much happened today.

When I arrived Drew waved his unique wave at me. When I asked how he was, he blew me away by replying "Pretty good, all things considered." He is becoming increasingly voluble and active. One of the nurses said, "He's wonderful, a real charmer." At this stage you might describe him as being like a happy drunk.

The nurses now must guard against his increased activity accidentally harming him.

Several times this afternoon Drew pushed himself into a sitting position to adjust his comfort or to make it easier to cough. However, he lacks balance due to the fact that his vision has not yet returned, his head injury and lying in bed for two weeks. He could easily fall over and further injure his head.

Tomorrow they will use a camera to check to make certain that he can swallow properly before they decide to remove the feeding tube. They are also going to try to get him sitting on the side of the bed with nurses and/or physiotherapists on each side of him.

His heart rate is still elevated but his pneumonia seems to have gone.

It has been a remarkable 48 hours. To underscore that, the doctor who was in charge of emergency when Drew was brought in was in ICU today and was overheard saying, "I didn't expect him to be here."

When Drew's mother, Rachel, left tonight, Drew tried to kiss her goodbye, in spite of the oxygen mask and wrist restraints.

Today I read him some of your recent postings. He was quite pleased and surprised to hear that you are all out there concerned about him and cheering him on.

16:D Drew sees & waves, "higher neural function school", higher motor skills signalling - Word is "party"
Wednesday, April 23 – evening

Drew was put onto a special "chair" this afternoon. Neil stood beside him and they seemed to be deeply engrossed in conversation as the two of them often get. Now conversation is a lot of work for both because it is often difficult to understand what Drew is saying for reasons I mentioned previously.

I stood 10 feet away asking his nurse, Nathalie, a question. As she replied in detail I looked at Drew and Neil. Drew was facing me. Even though I knew that his sight had not returned, for some reason I waved at him. He waved back. I was dumbfounded; he saw me wave!

While we knew that one eye had been responding to the nurse's flashlight, we had no previous indication that he could see. His "good" eye still is swollen shut. It is tempting to think that he saw me with his "bad" eye but we can't yet rule out that his good eye's lid had opened just a bit. Why not just ask him? Some things he can't answer; his mind may be in the warehouse taking inventory and he will answer with the closest relevant reply not necessarily the accurate reply. This will normalize in time. Therefore, as of yet we have no idea how well he can see or how well he will eventually be able to see.

The doctor in charge of the ICU today, Doctor Andrew Baker, had been in charge of the ICU the day after Drew was admitted and at that time had given us the straight goods, removing from us any expectations. Focusing us on the "now" was the kind of anaesthetic our emotions needed. Today he agreed that Drew had substantially exceeded expectations. He said that Drew would be sent to the "higher neural function school" which he explained was not really a school but a category for those who stood a good chance of returning to normal.

He also said that Drew's brain was no longer "hot", that is, vulnerable to further damage if for some reason he developed a fever. Even so, he said, they won't do the final neurosurgery for another two months or so once everything has settled down.

Prior to the wave, Nathalie had been explaining to me that what Drew had just gestured to Neil with both hands, the salute with the first and fourth finger extended, and the 2nd and 3rd closed, while saying to Neil "party", was an indication that he had his fine

43

motor skills, the highest level of physical functioning. She added that the gross motor skills, such as walking, somewhat weakened due to prolonged bed stay, would be brought back through physio.

On the whole, today, as yesterday, he was subdued but no longer sedated. He got a burst of energy when first sitting up talking to Neil. The Doctor Drew explained that these alternating cycles of lethargy and activity were quite normal.

He still has much to overcome. But Drew's word for today is "party".

Note: Today a phone call got through to me from a close family friend since Rachel's childhood, as are many of his brothers and sisters. Technology challenged, initially they hadn't been reading the Facebook postings so I provided a very brief overview. When he asked, "When can you and Rachel get together with us?" I replied, "Maybe in a year."

19:D Teleported to Gold Coast; age of parents; parallel processing
Thursday, April 24 – evening

Drew said that he thought that he'd been "teleported to a research facility." When asked where the hospital is that he is in, he said "Australia. The Gold Coast." When asked the same question the other night he said, "I haven't got a damn idea."

Clearly he has not pulled it all together yet but he is trying. This provides a variety of moments.

This evening he asked us, his parents, our ages. When we told him, he said, "Holy crap!"

It made us feel better when he said the same thing when we told him his age.

While bits and pieces of the recent past surface, he is most comfortable before 1999.

His short term memory is still not at all good. Stimulating it into action is one of the purposes of repeatedly asking him where he is and then telling him when he gets it wrong.

On the other hand he talked on for 5 minutes about "parallel processing" and how we allow over analyzing to add to the burden of useless information that inundates the margins of our lives. I kid you not. He had this discussion with a male nurse, Irwin, who has children aged 13 and 15 and likes Brian Enos and the Amon Tobin that was playing. Drew told Irwin, "Your kids are just embracing life. That was a good time for me. When can we talk about them again?" "Sunday", Irwin said."

Dr. Baker told us today that Drew is on a great recovery trajectory and that we should see significant progress over the next two weeks before the rate of progress diminishes. He said that Drew will be moved out of ICU for some months and then moved to a rehabilitation facility.

Drew launched into a discussion about the similarity between computational inputs and output systems being one system and that his feeding tube, IV and catheter were essentially the same thing, "really pretty simple systems," he said. Then he said, "who is that in blue?" I turned around to see a blue-jacketed nurse retreating around a corner about 20 feet away. "What was she dragging?" he said. Then he answered his own question, "It looked like a mop and pail." That would have been my guess too. His eyesight is better than I had expected.

I told him that you lot were looking forward to hearing the music that he would create after this experience. "Cool". "I can see lyrics and then riffs building on them, then more riffs. All of it organic. But I think that I'll let it play around inside for awhile first."

These are a few fragments of our discussion which lasted nearly an hour. For the rest of the day I understand that he slept or was prodded by physio, nurses and Doctors.

22 : D Drew Reads, zombie walk
Saturday, April 27 – evening

Anna Pfuller of Ottawa wins the bragging rights because her Saturday posting was the first one that Drew read. We knew that his vision was getting better but had no idea that he could yet read. We were blown away…

With his Aunt Marie, I stood by as two nurses got Drew standing to take just his second walk. Pretending to be a Zombie, he took his first steps towards his Aunt. His Zombie persona was shockingly realistic considering recent events and the condition that he is in. Then he hugged Marie. It was brilliant timing and couldn't have been scripted any better, taking us from shock to laughter to aaahh in seconds…

The staff disconnected him from all monitors today. … Drew is no longer critical but still requires 24/7 attention since his current lack of short term memory means that he doesn't remember what his weaknesses and vulnerabilities are and therefore he could inadvertently seriously injure himself. He is constantly trying to climb out of bed and would definitely fall if he did so unassisted…

Note: For me, his zombie shtick was a strong instance of the presence of the healthy, non-corporeal Drew. With his brain in its damaged condition three weeks after his injury, he should not have been able to conceive and carry off that joke. At the time I sensed his presence strongly; again healthy and separate from his damage-limited body and mind.

28 : D Smoking
Saturday, May 3 – morning

…

Along that line, one inadvertent benefit of his injury is that he has definitely quit smoking…

As a footnote to that, you would not believe the ugly crap they suctioned from his lungs during the first weeks he was in hospital even after he started coughing on his own. The Doctors and nurses told us from the beginning that smokers inevitably get pneumonia post-surgery or while in a coma. Drew had pneumonia 2, possibly 3 times. He was treated with massive doses of antibiotics all 3 times and developed an allergic reaction twice which drove up his temperature to the limit, more than doubled his heart rate exhausting him and covered his body in a rash. The high temperature prevented his brain swelling from improving. The nurses described the energy consumption of the high heart rate for 48 hours as equivalent to running a marathon for two days. Pneumonia not only could end the lives of such patients but also it plus the treatment deprives the body of the energy that it needs to heal.

Nothing quite focuses one's judgements about such matters as sitting for hours on end holding a loved one's hand, watching the minute by minute changes in the only other indications of life which were the digital and dynamic graphical readouts of heart rate, pulse rate, several different blood pressure readings, brain pressure, respirations per minute, and blood oxygen levels. It was literally as hands on as 36 hours of ICU nurses and family pushing his stomach up against his diaphragm to get him to breathe and repeating, "Drew your respiration has dropped below 7. Breathe deeply, let's get it over 10. That's it. Breathe deeply like you're playing the oboe again. Cough Drew. Cough."

The various specialists are assessing him…We have heard that the final neurosurgery may be farther off than had previously been suggested. The therapists responsible for his intellectual and emotional recovery are giving us an idea of what they will be doing with Drew, and helping us with advice, exercises that we should do with him, and various dos and don'ts for us. …

Drew finds life confusing at times. Particularly when he is tired, words don't come or are inappropriately applied as the result of "confabulation". It must be hard for the one who is accidentally confabulating, particularly if they don't realize that is what is happening and their mind is now cluttered with two words and two meanings where only one is the maximum Drew requires. It is frustrating to most when they can't recall a term, or someone's name doesn't come when they need it. That is but an annoyance compared to what Drew is living at the moment. But this phase too will pass. In the meantime it contributes to his exhaustion.

As a result we are learning a whole new patience repertoire, which I hope will payoff in other relationships as well, about which some of you will be glad to read!

Note: Doctors, nurses, and other professionals counselled us on the new reality of the injured brain. One said, "Once he has healed, think of his condition as similar to having had five concussions." They warned that tobacco, alcohol and recreational drugs as well as self-medicating were now banned for life. All of these would risk his brain health, brain function, emotions, and judgments. Eventually he could travel by airplane but he shouldn't ride a bike or do anything that risked banging his head. A sixth concussion could be fatal or permanently brain-altering. That advice changed all our lives for the short and long term. Drew had a number of food allergies, specifically to corn and grapes, which meant that he hardly ever touched beer or wine in any case. But we were mindful of the consequences of serving alcohol at family meals and while entertaining, particularly once he was recovering at home.

Now nearly 4-years after his accident, he takes an occasional quarter glass of wine and we know that he has reverted to going out for a smoke a few times a day. What do we do? Well, what can or should we do? He is 36. He knows we prefer that he did neither; although we say nothing. Very occasionally I have even poured him a requested partial glass of wine, if the rest of us are having wine with dinner. We are reassured knowing that he indulges in quantities that are far less than any other smoker or drinker. It is important that he make his own choices and self-regulate. It is important that he have normalcy and not be made to feel different.

1 : M
1 : D

Police, 50% cardio vascular, 20% of their muscle mass and 10% of their bone density; Drew on the floor
Tuesday, May 6 – evening

"What are you guys doing here?" a friendly Drew asked one of the two uniformed policemen sitting outside his door 24/7 for a week.

"Baby sitting your roommate," said one of them referring to a very quiet, polite, heavily tattooed guy chained to his bed...

In spite of these conversations, the semi-private room, to which Drew was moved down the hall from ICU, is quieter than ICU and Drew has been sleeping quite a bit the more that he is being exercised physically, verbally and intellectually. Now he can walk without support although accompanied.

His exercises are important for a significant number of reasons including short term memory through physical orientation and engaging all the senses, and for physical reconditioning. A Doctor explained that for anyone spending two weeks in a coma, they calculate that they have lost 50% of their cardio-vascular conditioning, 20% of their muscle mass and 10% of their bone density.

He still has a 24/7 "sitter" in part because he is still removing frequently the hard collar protecting his fractured vertebraee. It is not hard to understand why. However, in the discussion with him about why he needs to put it back on we get into circular discussion about the collar and a microphone. ...

1 : M
5 : D

2, 4, 24, 48 Vision; First time sees damage in a mirror
Saturday, May 10 – evening

"Two fingers. Now four fingers. I don't see them clearly, but I see them," said Drew uncovering his "good" left eye. Friday he revealed to Neil and Rachel that his right eye had regained some vision. Of course, I had to test him for myself. It was a thrill that I couldn't pass up.

Even having some, occasional vision in his right eye will give him some help with neuroplasticity, and some capacity for depth perception, important for walking, driving, balance and even kissing as Drew discovered through an abrupt stop. …

In the mirror he looked at the incision tilting his head down and side to side to get a better look at it through the hair that is growing back. "That looks pretty major," he said soberly. "It is Drew. You nearly died," I said. "No way," he said quietly. "Yes," I said, "You did." Now that his short term memory is improving he will be coming to terms with that reality. Perhaps it is best that his short term memory problem has dictated that he slowly remembers a bit more each time. …

Note: During the following days Drew repeatedly asked me how he came to be injured. I always replied, "We don't really know." Later that week, I told him that it was possible that he had been hit by a train but that we didn't know for certain. The next day, when he asked me, "Could I have done it?" I replied, "We don't know". I was grateful that the hospital psychologist, with whom the family had met, had told us to let Drew come to us with his memories or awareness of any desire or attempt to self-harm.

Neuroplasticity, referenced above, is the ability of the brain to rewire itself so that people can function as before even though part of their brain may be impaired. If you are interested in neuroplasticity there is a great optimism-making Penguin book by Dr. Norman Doidge, of the University of Toronto, titled *The Brain That Changes Itself*. The book was on the New York Times Best Seller list. Also, read My *Stroke of Insight* by Dr. Jill Bolte Taylor. There are wonderful on-line videos by and about both. Hospitals also have very informative resource materials describing what to expect at each step of recovery. See the *Appendices* for more information.

1 : M
6 : D

Mother's Day – Meltdown
Sunday, May 11 - Journal

Rachel and I took a break and walked a block into the Eaton Centre, out of the hospital for lunch for the first time. Later in the day, we were going to order in food to the hospital and the family would find a quiet place in the hospital to celebrate Mother's Day. The stimulation and noise at the Eaton Centre food court was overwhelming, battering our senses. We fled. A half block back to the hospital, Rachel had a loud, angry meltdown on the sidewalk in front of Massey Hall. This compounded my own distress but I got her back to the hospital. An hour or so later, I decided that I couldn't cope with being with our family which was about to arrive to celebrate Mother's Day and so I began to drive home. Rachel would spend the night at her sister's, which she had been doing for weeks because it was closer to the hospital.

When Neil phoned, I realized that I had been driving inattentively, automatically and somewhat aimlessly. I found myself driving towards where Drew was injured, not in a straight line towards home. Neil talked me back to the hospital. I didn't stay long; then went home where I stayed for two days.

Yes, watch for the emotional dominoes. Imploding or exploding is natural and necessary to release stress. However at each incident, someone else may have to control his or her stress in order to step in to contain and manage the patient's situation. Each pays a toll for that. Be ready for your turn.

1 : M
8 : D

Meditations
Sunday, May 13 - evening

"Your breath smells," said Drew Sunday. He had a headache and when I was cooling his forehead with my hand he covered his nose and mouth. I had asked him why. That was the third time that he had made the same comment over the previous 10 days. Naturally I was annoyed; I rather like Tim Hortons' coffee. But he had a right to his opinion. I wondered if his comments were due to the lack of inhibition due to the frontal lobe injury or if the injury had given him an acute sense of smell.

But I had asked him why he covered his nose? He said, "Because I didn't want to upset you." Very interesting, I thought. Drew must be redeveloping his sense of inhibition, a further sign of the healing of his brain.

… Drew's discussions are more and more apt for a greater part of the time. His Webbnet colleague and great friend visited and spoke at length with Drew about the office and colleagues and technology and, to paraphrase his friend, was very pleasantly surprised that Drew was almost totally like the old Drew.

… As we have experienced and seen in others at the hospital, the Drews of such traumas are not the only injuries. Drew is now leading some of us in recovery. His recovery has no imposed constraints. It is uninhibited. It has no emotional baggage waiting to sabotage it although he is coming to terms with the seriousness of what happened to him. …

Note: While Drew's sense of smell may not seem important, since he did not have a great sense of smell or taste before his injury, his surprising improvement in both areas was remarkable. We never did determine how much of this was due to his brain's changed condition and how much was due to the fact that he was no longer smoking. His chemoreceptor improvement is just one example of many possible patient-specific changes in perception, physiological response, or intellectual performance that you may notice due to the brain's changed state. Since some of them are positive, I find it difficult to choose an accurate descriptor. *Injured* and *traumatized* aren't accurate here and don't seem to be comprehensive enough.

In retrospect that Sunday Drew made a far more important comment. While at the time I was quite surprised and impressed by the remark to his visiting friend, only 4 years later did I realize that his comment has shaped fundamentally my own attitude to Drew and to all others—not just the injured. Thirty-eight days after his pierced and dramatically swollen brain seemed to doctors to be too damaged to support life, Drew's brain decided that, "I'm not worse nor better; just different." Since then, and even more strongly now, that phrase comes unbidden to mediate my responses to others. Slowly this process weeds out not-so-nice ingrained responses.

Listen to the patient; there is wisdom there. But, it may be up to you to make it visible to others, including the patient.

1:M 14:D Off medications, Roommates, "Hope" stone
Monday, May 19 – morning

…Last week they took him off the last major medications: anti-coagulants, and medicines for lowering his heart rate and for anxiety. As a result he is often serious, occasionally argumentative in a nice way. The collar continues to be a reoccurring subject of discussion, and increasingly, the fact that he must always be accompanied any time he gets out of bed.

Now he asks questions, sometimes not wanting to know the complete answer: what is the risk of fractured vertebraee; what are the specifics of the damage to his skull and brain; what were the stages of his recovery. He said that he wishes that he could remember. I said that I wished that I could forget. Neither of us were completely accurate. I broke the subsequent reflective silence to remind us both that what has happened is not nearly as important as what lies ahead. I suggested to Drew that should he never know the specifics, he should be satisfied with the two miracles he experienced: survival, and his amazing ongoing recovery. But to know Drew is to know intense curiosity and he seems tired and even anxious as he forces his not yet healed brain to resolve this so that he can be at peace with it.

Drew told me that his brother JJ, a strong, ex-ocean lifeguard at Myrtle Beach, accompanied Drew to the (special) shower last week to look after him. Apparently, JJ got into the spirit and was semi-naked, probably trying to cajole Drew along. They then took to laughing so hard that Drew developed a severe headache and had to return to bed and Tylenol 3. …

53

Note: Tonight we arrived home to find on our doorstep a 2-inch, semi-spherical, soapstone carving engraved with the word *Hope*. We still don't know who left it. It sits in our hall. Neighbours and strangers helped us in many ways including leaving flowers and meals on our doorstep once we were on a regular schedule. Drew's friends both brought snack food for us to the hospital in the first few days knowing that we would not be leaving the 9th floor. Another group paid for a $700 gift certificate for a service that allowed us to order meals from dozens of great restaurants in the region and to have the meals delivered to us at the hospital or at home.

Drew's first posting
Tuesday, May 20 – evening

1 : M
15 : D

See the posting on the Wall below at 8:56 tonight.

I'm one big grin.

Drew Powell (Toronto, ON) wrote at 8:56 pm on May 20th, 2008

Yah! I'm a little strange. I only got my consciousness in the past 7 days and have no memories of the past 50 days which I've been in hospital the entire time for. A little weird, but I'm rebuilding everything.

First time outside in 49 days - Hospital #3
Friday, May 23

1 : M
18 : D

Drew, a Securitas Guard (his current minder) and I went for a longish walk outside today and sat in a shaded arbour for 20 minutes. This is Drew's first time outside in 49 days. While passing the time we tested his bad right eye. He can't see much detail but he can see buildings, clouds, nearby people and vehicles and tell colour. His peripheral vision seems to be normal. … The shortcomings are such that if someone passes him from behind on his right he can be thrown off balance. …

Note: This third hospital was an interim step until a bed came available in a rehabilitation hospital.

1 : M
20 : D

Burning Man Thighs
Sunday, May 25 – morning

Drew is applying the name "burning man" to his thighs. Since Friday he has been walking a lot outside in the sun. As he builds strength his thighs are hurting and he is loving it. One of his Securitas minders is a practitioner of martial arts. He has been talking to Drew about strengthening himself by exercising through the burn. Interestingly, Drew is listening and adopting. He says that he is looking forward to his new physio regime.

He is also scaring his minders, and family, as he deliberately walks along curbs and across uneven lawns. He is deliberately testing his balance and his vision and doesn't always tell us beforehand.

He is teaching himself coping skills in addition to ones already introduced to him by the physio specialist who started him in ICU.
…

1 : M
23 : D

Walk in the woods, bone plate, arggh
Wednesday, May 28 – evening

This is a cautionary tale for those of you who meet with Drew one-on-one in the near term.

Today Drew put himself at risk. This afternoon he persuaded a first time visitor to walk with him in the woods behind the hospital. Drew "thought" it was low risk. The problem is that he is at that stage in his recovery where he cannot make such judgments even though he sounds completely rational and in command of the facts.

The reality is that his balance is impaired due to having spent so long in bed and due to the fact that his right eye has very poor vision. Consequently he lacks depth perception, can't easily read slopes or uneven ground, rocks or tree branches even in direct light never mind in the changing light qualities of a forest. Due to the bed rest, his muscles are not strong and if he were to stumble he would not be able to prevent himself from falling.

In taking this adventure, his recovering brain did not give sufficient weight to his extra vulnerability not only to falling but to re-injuring his brain given that: his brain is not yet healed; and his brain is not protected by the usual bone in his forehead and the left side of his skull, both of which have been temporarily removed to allow his brain to swell and then to return to normal. To think of a comparative vulnerability, think of an egg with 25% of the shell removed.

He can easily fall at any time although to date he has not. Imagine the results of even a "benign" fall given that he gets serious head pains from lying on his left side (which he is forbidden to do), sitting up too quickly or laughing or sneezing too hard. A fall in a hospital room or corridor with smooth walls is potentially damaging to him. However, this was a longish walk on uneven, littered ground through woods with sharp branches.

His judgments will improve and his vulnerabilities decrease with time. In the meantime, do him a big favour by not doing him any favours that don't seem right. A big tip off that something might not be OK is if you ask Drew if it is OK and he says that it is low risk! And be prepared for Drew to argue. Tell him that you are uncomfortable and that you are only protecting him. Keep a sense of humour in the face of his frustration. If you have any questions ask them at the nursing station and take Drew with you. He accepts what the professionals say.

It is a positive sign that Drew wants to push the envelope, take on greater responsibility for himself and get out in the world. It is positive that he wants to resume his life. His frustration is understandable as is his rediscovered joy of life.

But...aaargh!

Note: In this hospital we began to encounter serious conflicts of will. Drew demanded that we provide him with his wallet, his phone and his laptop, none of which he was in any condition to use. Furthermore, all hospitals strongly recommended that such items not be provided to any patient because they could be stolen. However, for Drew these must have been things that, in a primal way, he saw as indication that he was returning to normalcy. Unfortunately, he was nowhere near normal but his brain injuries were preventing him from making that judgment. The confrontations were becoming so unpleasant that, for some days we kept our visits to the bare minimum and then did not stay long. Eventually we did allow him to have his laptop but he found that he could not use it in a way that was satisfactory to him so we took it home.

Eventually, I admitted to throwing his wallet out, together with his bloody clothes in the first week.

2 : M
3 : D

Bridgepoint - Hospital #4
Visiting, Rehabilitation
June 8, Sunday – evening

As he wrote in a post to the Wall today, Drew is interested in people contacting him to set up visits. …

Drew has embraced this first week of rehab. He is enjoying the classes and those giving them. The change in him is noticeable. He is generally more content even as he pushes the limits of his classes, energy and some of the necessary restraints on him.

Ever since he began to speak he showed signs of being more eloquent and even more mature than before he was injured. This is in spite of still recovering from his injuries and manifesting some of the typical symptoms of Acquired Brain Injury (ABI) patients. His brain trauma has "rebooted" him in unforeseen ways, all positive, erasing some concerns and releasing new strengths.

Your proverbs, aphorisms, quotations and jokes about "patience" have been helpful to me, to us and perhaps even to Drew as well. …

In reflecting on his week, Drew mentioned his fellow patients and an observation about them and stories told him by the staff about past patients who have volunteered to help others with similar difficulties. Drew is already talking to staff about doing that himself.

I paraphrase and can't convey Drew's insight with anywhere near his eloquence. "Many people are closed up because their hearts have never been touched by strangers. Once you suffer a major injury you find yourself in the care of strangers, of people who are doing what they do because they care. This touches the patient's heart and so they become more outgoing and want to give back."

2:M 10:D Cluck Grunt and Low; first night out
Sunday, June 15

Cluck Grunt and Low was the restaurant where Drew, JJ and Neil took their father for Father's Day supper Sunday. Somehow it seemed fitting. The food was great and the yuks were many. Drew ate everything. For the whole weekend we were helping him regain the 25 pounds he has lost, 20% of his body weight.

Drew was quite at ease with his appearance (surgical collar, dark wrap around glasses and black hat with a bit of scar on his forehead showing) and the stares that he frequently gets.

This was the first time Drew had been out of the hospital overnight since April 5th. As weekends at home go it was pretty normal. …

Friday night we sat on the porch and watched the spectacular lightening and rain storm, something we always did with the boys. Saturday in particular was very relaxing. We walked and Drew talked to neighbours who have been very supportive over the recent months.

Sunday we visited Drew's loft where he helped us identify things that needed packing for the move expected this week. …

Sunday Rachel made a Father's Day brunch for the 3 of us. Having Drew home made this Father's Day the best.

3 : M
20 : D

Drew has been discharged from the hospital!
Webbnet party at the Docks
Friday, July 25 - Day 111

Drew was discharged from hospital on day 111 of his hospitalisation. He went directly to his Webbnet's office party at the DOCKS at Polson Pier with his father and Uncle Brian, visiting from Australia, in tow. Needless to say, it was a gloriously sunny summer's day.

Drew's reunion with his Webbnet's colleagues was emotional and joyous. He had been looking forward to it for a long time. It was wonderful to witness and I will post pictures below.

Drew is now living for some months at home with his parents in Richmond Hill while he continues 10-12 weeks of outpatient therapy 2-3 days a week. ...

At the Webbnet's party, after a group of colleagues excitedly hugged Drew and shook his hand, big grins all round, one colleague asked the resurrected Drew, "Well, what have you learned?"

After a few seconds, Drew replied, "It is good to be alive."

To which all seemed to reply, "Amen to that."

Note: Later that day Drew told me that he thought before answering. This is a sign of healing of his brain's frontal lobe. For quite some time, when people asked him what happened to him he would joke, "I kissed a train." They all went white in the face. I explained to Drew that while it was quite funny, in a black sort of way, other people were very upset by his joke. Furthermore, we did not know how he was injured, so joking about a train would confirm an inaccurate rumour.

4 : M
27 : D

DJd Cherry Beach today
Monday, September 1

Drew "Mental Floss" DJd Cherry Beach to day. This was his first gig since he was injured. Many friends turned out. Pictures will be posted below.

The family, along with Drew's friends celebrated Drew's 33rd birthday there as well. ...

It was a glorious summer day and a glorious event.

4 : M
16 : D

Drew DJd the Harvest Festival north of Huntsville
Sunday, September 21

Drew DJd the pyramid last night at the Harvest Festival north of Huntsville. ...

Drew had an exhilarating but very tiring day. He had been looking forward to Harvest for months. There was much Drew hugging from friends who had not seen him since before the accident.

Watching Drew DJ, one friend said, "Looking at him you can't tell that anything happened to him. It is amazing to see him here after what he has been through."

For JJ and my part, it was great to see Drew in his element and to meet so many of Drew's wonderful friends after having read their messages of love and encouragement over the past few months. ...

Note: If you can believe it, Drew had DJd an afternoon, outdoor, roller skating event the previous month, only four months after his injury. I had seen it as a dry run as Drew was absolutely determined to DJ this autumn, three-day, camping event for more than three hundred people as he had done for six years. Drew let us know for months that he intended to DJ this event but, in spite of his demands, I could not let him camp for the weekend even if I were to camp with him. From what I had been told, these were up-til-sunrise events. Drew did not have the energy to cope and would pay a painful price if he did not get enough rest.

I was prepared to let him make decisions where I was confident that he knew and appreciated the consequences, but I was not prepared to allow him to expose himself to high-risk vulnerability. I imagine that it was a grey area legally, but he seemed to have developed an evolving trust arrangement with his family, even if it was occasionally contentious as he drove his recovery. In this instance, I could not let him walk around in the pitch black night on uneven ground, in rock, tree and tent peg strewn fields with fifty percent of his protective skull missing. It made me sick to even briefly contemplate the consequences.

Very few of the partying campers had seen Drew since he had been injured. Although they had spoken to him, none of the event organizers had seen him and yet, sensitively, they agreed to schedule him into a DJing slot. As I came to learn, this was a partying community but first and foremost it was a community—they looked after and cared for each other like loved family.

Knowing what was at stake, both positively and negatively, I did not mind the long drive up and back the same day. I was very glad that JJ volunteered to share the driving, and to participate in the experience which he could then recount to our family.

I was becoming Drew's driver, roadie and bodyguard for such events. That night in the large pyramid tent, JJ and I were compelled to dance, party and be hugged by Drew's many attractive friends. It was awful! I was twenty-five again! Drew was my "get out of jail card" for many such events, for which I will always be grateful to him. Seeing the joyfully tearful reception that Drew received from his friends and getting to know them at such events, and through the Facebook postings from an even larger community, his family came to appreciate many wonderful new dimensions of Drew. JJ and I made many wonderful friends that night.

Drew ended up DJing longer than he was booked for because another DJ hadn't turned up. Well past midnight when Drew finished, he was incapacitated by both exhaustion and the resultant massive headaches that he experienced almost daily during the previous months. To return to the car, JJ and I had to hold Drew up as we walked him for 15 minutes in the dark, out of the bush over the uneven trails.

Drew knew in advance what he would be putting himself through. He reclined in the car, in great pain but very happy. This night was a huge psychological boost both for Drew and for his many supportive friends. Drew inspired us all.

I cannot over-emphasize how important this event was for Drew's re-validation. Setting and achieving such milestones are absolutely imperative for patient, family, friends, health-care professionals and employers. At the company's summer party on the day that Drew left hospital, the company president perceptively told me that holding Drew's job open for him would be an important milestone for Drew to work towards and to motivate his recovery.

That DJing event in the bush took some of the self-imposed pressure off Drew to validate himself. It was an important sign that he was recovering his life and it was, also, an important reminder of his limits at that stage of his recovery. Two other self-validation milestones remained: return to work and return to independent living.

5:M
23:D

Therapy routine
September 28 - Journal

Drew made great strides with his therapists. He was still an outpatient so Rachel drove Drew to nearly all of his appointments and I drove him to some. Drive 40 kilometres; wait 1-4 hours; turn around and drive home again. We didn't begrudge doing it but still it was an inconvenient grind, and expensive in time and money.

While he was grateful that we took him to his appointments, he was eager to gain his independence. For us all, that would be a marker for healing and ability to undertake some degree of self-responsibility.

One of the therapists' tasks was to ensure that Drew would be safe taking public transit. To start they would have Drew plan an outing which they took together, the therapist controlling the agenda and monitoring Drew's behaviour, attention, orientation, balance and safety consciousness. Then they had Drew plan and lead as they travelled the route. Finally, they would send him off on his own, following and observing him at a distance. From our home, he had to take a regional bus plus the subway or GO Transit train plus a streetcar. It was a challenge but he was making progress towards some degree of independence and the required mental state that permitted him to do that safely.

The therapists approved Drew to travel from home to the hospital for therapy and medical appointments. Quite naturally, Rachel was all for Drew removing from her some of the necessity of driving and waiting, even if in the beginning he would get himself to his half-day of appointments and then one of us would drive down and pick him up.

When I heard this I said to the therapist and Rachel together that Drew would not be travelling on this own very soon even if he had the skills to do so. "Why not?" they asked. I replied, "Because the consequences if he is banged, or falls are far too great." "How so?" they asked. I answered, "Think of it this way. Think of how strong an egg is. Now think of how much weaker it is once you remove 50% of the shell. The rest of the shell will crack much more easily. As it is, the front half of his brain has absolutely no protection should he fall forward. A sharp object such as someone's back pack could puncture his brain. If he falls backward, the skull that is there no longer has its integrity and would crack easily.

They hadn't thought of that. Then I mentioned the "strap of death".

Drew would leave home to go on public transit, with us or his therapist, always carrying a large backpack with his stuff. Inevitably, there was strap hanging down. Having been safety trained at my student summer jobs in factories and on construction sites, I was concerned that the strap would snag on something that would make him fall or bang his head, or worse still, catch in something moving such as an escalator or subway car he was exiting. I told him this. He was not pleased and obviously thought that it was not a risk. I started referring to it as the "strap of death".

His answer at such times was often, "Well I've been doing it for years and nothing serious has happened!" I replied, "That was then. Your risk now, should the unlikely happen, is tremendously greater. Before, if you fell you might get a cut or a bump on the head. Now there is nothing between your brain and any blunt or sharp object. Furthermore, your brain is still injured and still healing. What would have been a nasty experience before, could be fatal now." We continued using this description until he got the point and began to fasten the strap or tuck it in. His mother and his therapists also had words with him about it. Eventually, we felt that he was sufficiently situationally aware that he could travel on his own if he weren't tired. One of the major consequences of brain injury is years of exceptional fatigue.

When he was tired, the drives to and from appointments could be interestingly conversational, briefly confrontational or we listened to the radio. After all, what we were experiencing was the *teenage years* of his recovery. We did not begrudge the time together, whatever the quality.

Progress is a mixture of healing, determination, support, good therapists (physio, psycho, occupational) and time. Your timetable is relative; it is not fixed. We had already accepted that where Drew is at any stage may be where he may be for the rest of his life. Any progress was welcome but not necessary.

Progress came unannounced. If you weren't listening you may not have noticed. You suddenly realize, "something has changed." Then we tried to figure out what. Often the progress that we noticed was in social interaction, personality—subtle things.

6 : M DJing, roller-skating and public scrutiny
Sunday October 5 - Journal

Drew DJd a roller-skating party at an outdoor municipal rink. Mr. *Uninhibited* had a great time talking to people, many of whom had heard about his injury but had not seen him since his accident. I went along as his roadie and driver. I gained an additional title there.

As Drew DJd, I noted that the speeding roller skaters, some of them quite unsteady, came along an arc towards his DJ table. Then, eight feet away, they turned. If one were to falter mid-turn, there was nothing to prevent them from crashing into Drew but his light DJ-equipment table. I positioned myself to be able to see skaters coming towards him in order to be able to grab him out of the way if there was any risk.

At one point, an attractive young woman, walked up to Drew to talk with him as he DJd. Suddenly, a very large wasp landed on Drew's forehead, his stinger only a quarter inch of skin away from Drew's brain. I launched myself over six feet at Drew, removing the determined wasp. Drew was quite matter of fact about it; his friend was a little shaken. Minutes later she said to me, "Is this what you do? Security for Drew?"

Not quite getting her meaning, I replied, flippantly, "Well the groupies haven't been bad yet." Then it dawned on me that what Drew and our family took as normal, must appear to others to be quite unusual. His appearance for starters, initially with wide-open, wandering right eye, a scarred, sloping forehead and a surgical collar, then with a black toque-like hat knit by a former girlfriend. Also, he travelled with this guy who was obviously far older than anyone else there and who turned out to be his father.

We took our cue from Drew when it came to subjecting him to scrutiny in public places. Had I been him, likely I would have avoided unnecessary embarrassing scrutiny. One day while he was an in-patient, but allowed to leave the rehabilitation hospital when escorted, Drew, Neil and I walked chatting up to *Allen's*

Restaurant on Danforth Avenue to have lunch in the sunny back patio. Allen's is a nice, casual, somewhat upscale Irish New York saloon style restaurant typical of and historically connected through its design and its proprietor to Allen's restaurant in New York. Drew was aware but not self-conscious at having others stare at him. If he was OK with it, who were we to be self-conscious? Furthermore, this was the worst that he would look and so if he could cope with that here then he could cope anywhere with whatever he would eventually look like.

To what extent his lack of obvious discomfort was the result of his judgment or his lack of inhibition due to his injured frontal lobe, we will never know. I do know that today looking at pictures we took of that first public lunch in Allen's patio, and seeing what I took for normal then, makes me both awestruck and slightly queasy. It was Drew's courage that accompanied us through it and many other similar events. He was becoming the "accompanyer".

5 : M + Meetings and dialogues with Drew's doctors, Bridgepoint Rehabilitation Hospital therapists and his psychotherapist

The Doctors' and therapists' legal and professional responsibility was to Drew not to us, even though we were Drew's guardian. However, they included us as part of the caregiver team as we appeared to be reasonable people, not in a hurry and not asking for miracles. They also knew that we would work the system on Drew's behalf if we felt that he weren't getting the professional service that he needed. They respected that.

Deliberately we established strong personal relationships with them all. In the beginning there were many reasons for us to attend the consultations, not the least of which was Drew's iffy ability to comprehend both what they said and what he said, on any given day. We were quasi-translators, note takers and appointment makers. Occasionally, we would brief the Doctors on his state of mind, either beforehand or in the meeting. Drew accepted our role as necessary and in his best interests, in part, because we accepted that we were unofficial parties and because we pre-empted problems where we could. One example was the ophthalmological surgeon dealing with Drew's bad eye. There were a number of medical procedures about which Drew could be squeamish, although the accident and subsequent months of treatment diminished those significantly. But I was concerned that Drew might react negatively to the suggestion that he would be awake when they conducted the short, out-patient surgery that straightened his eye and so alerted the Doctor in advance. He handled Drew perfectly and Drew approved going ahead with the procedure.

Even after Drew's first few sessions with the private psychotherapist that we attended, we, his parents, maintained dialogue with the psychotherapist. Drew knew this. Where we observed things that might need attention we would meet with her or email her. After all, at most she would see him once a week in her office. She wasn't around him 24/7. While he was trusting, fully disclosing, honest and forthright with her about his life, he was seeing it from within his healing perceptions. We were trying to be objective and trying to understand.

With Drew we had our good days and our bad days. We had our conflicts as any family does. Drew had always had strong likes and dislikes; strong focus on what interested him; strong desire to bend the world to his preferences. You won't be surprised to learn that he shared some of these characteristics, in some degrees, with his parents. Occasional conflict was inevitable. We were all take-charge people which could be read not as trying to fix something according to how we saw the world, but as meddling, interfering or just boring. Admittedly we weren't perfect—some of the time.

Both causing and over-riding this occasional friction was our desire for Drew to become the strongest person that he could. Eventually he would leave home again. We wanted to know that he would be able to take care of himself and, eventually, a family; that he would flourish; be successful and happy.

We had to let go progressively; let him take on increasing responsibilities, imperfectly to start. Fail and succeed.

We too failed, succeeded and improved. Drew and his psychotherapist, Ramona, taught us a great deal step by step. Drew progressed but so did we.

Years ago Drew labelled my occasional propensity for over-explaining as "kicking the flywheel". The heavy flywheel in an engine stores kinetic energy and, thereby, enables the idling heavy vehicle or industrial machine to come back up to speed quickly and with force. So a flywheel in an engine is a good thing; in your father—not so much. Drew always picked up things faster than I gave him credit for. Now I had to calibrate what I said to his frequently changing mental state and I didn't always get it right. But he made the situation worse because rather than acknowledge in some way that he had heard and understood, even though he might not agree, he would blow me off. Not the right thing to do to slow the flywheel down, it just energized it more. This became, in his eyes, a conflict of wills. In my eyes, I thought that I was being objective and did not have a vested interest in being right. I just wanted him to learn or to refute what I was saying, or take it under advisement, etc. Naturally it led to conflict and Ramona helped us both work it through.

It didn't help that he refused to acknowledge that there was such a thing as objectivity versus subjectivity. That made me very concerned that to go through life like that would leave him vulnerable. I have spoken to a number of psychologists about that subject and they have told me that there are people who cannot see the difference. It is not a matter of wilfulness or lack of education or experience. They cannot comprehend the distinction. In this regard, they cannot walk and chew gum. I saw this as setting him up for future conflict.

6 : M
2 : D

Seeking photographs for reconstructive surgery
Wednesday, October 7

We are looking for your help for Drew. As you will recall, Drew's bone plate surgery will happen within the next month. The surgeons want a few high quality images of Drew's forehead from his pre-injury days.

We need high quality, high resolution images of Drew's face with his forehead visible. Such pictures probably would come from his pony tail days. We need left and right profiles and frontal. We need to be able to print the pictures to 8x10. …

8 : M
12 : D

Drew has surgery
December 17 - Journal

Neurosurgeons and plastic surgeons reassembled Drew's skull from many of his bone fragments, titanium and polycarbonates. He overnighted in NeuroTrauma ICU where many of the staff were thrilled to see one of their former patients having progressed so well, something that, sadly, they seldom get to see.

9 : M
3 : D

Funeral of great aunt
January 8 - Journal

Drew attended the funeral and wake for a much-loved elderly Aunt who was definitely a character. She would have found it appropriate that Drew attended with his post-surgery short hair, and other dramatic signs of his still healing skull, including lines of staples across his forehead and down one side. He was quite matter of fact about it; but some of those attending   not so much. He talked to people during the entire wake. It matters not that his attitude was probably a combination of the still healing frontal lobe, which controls inhibition, and his own determination. The benefits to him far outweighed any down side. This was a judgment call that we let him make, as we were doing more and more.

17:M
10:D

Return to work
September 15

Today Drew returned to work at Webbnet to great jubilation.
Plants placed on his desk and lovingly tended from his first day of
absence were there to greet him.

20:M
16:D

Surgery successful
December 21

Drew's surgery went well. He is expected out of the hospital
tomorrow. It was wonderful for Drew, us and many of the staff in
the St. Michael's Hospital NeuroTrauma ICU to have a reunion.
They said that they were very happy and grateful as they seldom
get to see such a miraculous recovery of someone whose life had
been in their hands.

22:M
11:D

Drew's recovery & return to work is validated!
Wednesday, February 17

You will recall that we were told that the Monday after Drew was
injured, news of his life-threatening injury brought the company
to a virtual standstill.

Only six months ago, September 15, Drew started back to work,
moving progressively as his healing permitted up to the current 3
full-time days per week. For the past few months Drew has been
assigned the task of re-writing and organizing the web site that
Webbnet uses to communicate with its global user base. The
web site was then to be moved to a new server. While Drew, his
therapists and the Webbnet personnel worked to integrate Drew
successfully back into the company it was somewhat of an act of
faith for them to assign him a job of such importance to
the company.

Tuesday it went live. Today Drew received all kinds of accolades
from his colleagues and Webbnet executives. The site worked
well. They were happy for that but it sounds like most of all they

were happy for Drew. As a result, Drew has been beaming with a glow of joy. So have we. This event has been an unexpected gift.

For the first time Drew was able to walk around the company and talk to his colleagues about something that he had done which they could see and evaluate, and he could enlist their help to find ways to make it even better.

This launch is the first concrete indication for anyone, including Drew, of just of how well Drew has recovered intellectually and how capable he is in his new position. It is a huge validation milestone for everyone, for their individual and collective efforts. Of course Drew deserves the most credit for he has been amazingly determined, focused, and unrelentingly hard working. He has worked assiduously not only on regaining his technical competence but also on his inter-personal and team skills. He has been determined to come out of this better than ever.

I dithered about posting this but two things persuaded me to do so. It is great news, that Drew would be reticent about posting. Furthermore, we owe you the right to share in it. Each in your own way have provided important support for Drew therefore enjoy this milestone.

Drew is currently working 3 full-time days and in six weeks or so will be increasing that to 5 full-time days. There are still more objectives to check off but Drew is on the final leg of his journey.

23:M 19:D

Surgery
March 24 - evening

Posting retroactively deleted. For the reason, see the Journal entry below at page 75.

23:M
20:D

Surgeon's report
March 25 - 9:46 PM

The plastic surgeon told me that all went well during the 3-hour procedure and that Drew will be discharged and come home Friday.

When we left Drew at 8 tonight he was talking, walking and returning to his pre-anaesthetized self. He was particularly galvanized into life by the nurse mentioning one word - "catheter".

There is what looks like Scotch tape across his forehead, some swelling and a few other indicators but we expect that within two weeks no one will be able to notice anything, unless Drew provides a tour, as he is often willing to do. You know, once a techie always a techie…

Note: You will recall that the Day 1 emergency surgery removed fifty-percent of Drew's skull, from the top of his head down to his ears and forward to his eyebrows. The many bone fragments that they removed were stored using a process only developed in recent years. A critical part of the storage process for such bones is to keep them vital and viable for eventual re-construction. For this reason, sometimes the fragments are stored in the body cavity. Some of Drew's bone fragments were too damaged or non-viable to be reused and were replaced with a combination of metal and plastic. All these parts were held together by titanium screws. However, six months after the cranioplastic surgery re-established Drew's skull, developing indentations in his forehead indicated that the assemblage was not working. Imaging confirmed this. Some of the bone fragments were no longer viable. This fourth surgery replaced some of the skull with a shaped polymer skull plate. Primarily, this was done for structural integrity reasons but it also provided cosmetic benefits.

On his lap top, Drew has copies of the 3D imaging of his head which he shows enthusiastically to others to prove a point—with reactions varying from blanching to intense curiosity. His good humour and unemotional technical interest in the procedures has endeared him to all of his surgeons.

23:M 22:D Surgery over
March 26 - 4:22 PM

Drew came home at noon Friday. He is doing quite well; he has been over-energized since this morning. I imagine that he is on-line and reachable. It will take some time to work the anaesthetic out of his system and I imagine that he will have an energy crash in the next couple of days. So give him time if he doesn't seem to be completely himself.

23:M 22:D Irregularities and the Sacks of Dread
March 19-31 - Journal

Remember the Sack of Dread? I had thought that it had gone. In reality the body asserts its authority, sometimes unexpectedly. Related and unrelated matters, even good news can leverage our vulnerabilities. Also, our respective Sacks are by no means synchronized with each other. Any one of us can react or do instinctive things, sometimes in spite of our better judgment that, unwittingly, can trigger ruptures for others, creating an unintended ugly cascade of consequences.

Late in the afternoon of the day before the surgery, I had dropped Rachel and Drew at St. Mike's for the admission process and I made use of my invitation to a CBC-TV reception. It preceded the official screening of episode one of the TV miniseries *Keep Your Head Up, Kid: The Don Cherry Story*. Given the rough and tumble type of hockey that Cherry promotes and the subsequent discussion of debilitating hockey concussions, even more now than then I see going to this event as an odd choice of ways to pass the time the night before Drew's cranioplasty. The producer, a good friend, had invited me. He introduced me to Don Cherry and other cast members. My friend's wife and adult sons whom I had known a long time were there and I had a good time catching up with them and meeting a variety of personable broadcast celebrities. It was just what I needed to distract me. An hour into the event, Rachel called to say that Drew was through the admission process and they were at the hospital coffee shop for a snack, his last food until after his surgery. I left the reception immediately to join them.

As I exited the CBC elevator, I received a call from the Toronto police. The words and intonation sucked me back two years into that Saturday noon. It disoriented me; I had to sit down.

A few days before, the manager of the long-term care facility that looked after Rachel's ninety-two-year-old mother phoned. He reported that he suspected that her mother had suffered elder abuse by one of his staff. The manager wanted to get to the bottom of it but Rachel's mother, a strong-willed, take-charge, former senior nurse, was not volunteering any information. He wanted Rachel to be present when he questioned her mother so that he could collect the evidence that he needed to discipline, fire or even charge the offending staff member. That call compounded Rachel's stress—already high.

Rachel assured herself that the manager had already parked the suspect staff member somewhere safe and permanently away from her mother. Rachel had met, liked and trusted the manager but she also realised that he was in a conflict of interest.

Rachel's stress diminished somewhat when she spoke to her mother who confirmed that she was not injured and, apparently, was in good spirits.

As much as she wanted to help the manager to collect evidence to justify removing the alleged elder abuser from contact with all vulnerable elderly, Rachel had already realised that questioning her mother was likely pointless. Rachel suspected that her strong-willed mother had already decided that the incident was over and she didn't want further involvement.

Rachel explained Drew's surgery to the manager and said that she would come for the questioning—after the surgery.

Apparently, the manager felt obligated, perhaps by law or regulation, to call the police in immediately. In reality, his decision was in the best interest of all concerned, particularly that of Rachel's mother and the other residents. The two policemen that arrived immediately to question Rachel's mother, one of whom was speaking with me on the phone, could pry nothing out of this sub-five-foot, ninety-two-year-old, strong-willed woman. No surprise in that. Even with her declining faculties, she determined that she was safe and therefore did not want to become involved in a lengthy process to prosecute the staff member. The officer explained that they needed our persuasive help or they couldn't proceed.

Shakily back in the present, on the way to the hospital I determined to keep this call to myself for the time being. This decision was reinforced at the hospital where Drew seemed quiet but fine and Rachel was quiet but tense.

Before going to bed early, I posted on Facebook that Drew was undergoing surgery and asked his friends to give him some supportive thought. Even as I felt compelled to make that posting and the subsequent two postings, I sensed that they were a mistake. Drew had told very few people that he was having surgery. I suspect that, quite reasonably, he wanted to transition into a life where people treated him as any other normal person and not as brain injured.

We arrived at the hospital the next morning at 7:45, half an hour ahead of his scheduled departure to surgery. There were Rachel, JJ, Neil, and me in this small room. While we had no reason to worry about the surgery and Drew was completely at peace with it, by the time Drew was wheeled to surgery ninety minutes late, all five of us were stressed. We stayed away from each other for several hours while we waited for one of our favourite surgeons, Dr. Mahoney, to appear and give us the "expected" good news, which he did.

At supper two days after he returned home, Drew told me that he was very upset that I had emailed all of the Facebook registrants that he was having surgery. Being somewhat of a techno-Luddite, I was unaware that my posting had been emailed out. We had a short emotional discussion. He asked me why I had posted anything. Without any thought, I blurted out tearfully, "Because I was afraid that you might die!"

For the next two weeks, I withdrew completely from family and friends. My family didn't believe me until unilaterally I emailed far-away, imminently-arriving great friends and told them that I was cancelling our scheduled, long overdue get-together. Then, for the first time ever, the family saw the need to cancel our annual Easter gathering.

During the following weeks, I would suddenly develop an elevated temperature and nausea. I slept a lot and took long vigorous walks two or three times a day to pre-empt stress. Even so, I had the sense that I was on the edge of something worse if I didn't deal with it. That was my most serious crash to date. A year later Drew told me that my crash had a major impact on him. We have not been able to discuss what that meant. Why not? Those Sacks of Dread. There are still many subjects that we can't discuss with each other, but we are adding fewer as time goes on.

Sixth surgery
January 25 - Journal

2 : Y
9 : M
20 : D

At 1 p.m., day 1026, at the door to the St. Michael's Operating Room, Drew's wonderful plastic surgeon, Dr. Mahoney, the hospital's senior plastic surgeon, told us that he could not get the hospital to extend his surgery time and that Drew's 6th surgery would have to be postponed, for the second time.

The surgeon told us that his first procedure of the day had gone three hours, twice as long as forecast. We should hear in the next few days when they will reschedule him early enough in the day so that he won't be bumped a third time.

Yes disappointing, but as Drew said, "Better the guy that needed the extra work gets Dr. Mahoney's time than me. I'm not an emergency." In retrospect, I sensed that the staff were gratified at how calm and loose we were—no stress, no tantrums.

This may surprise you but the day went by pretty much without any obvious stress. Drew and I actually had a good time together. Remember the *new normal?* Maybe we we're finally moving into the adult-friends relationship and away from the problematic father/son conflicts of the past.

The next day, we were both very tired. I was a little manic, unable to focus. I had an attack of the *budgies*, talking a lot about little which caused Drew and me to have a mild reoccurrence of our core conflict. Drew is becoming aware that he too must be a caregiver.

Sasha, our family's small, furry *therapy* dog—a Kerswill terrier— had it worst. Being dropped suddenly and inexplicably at a friend's house was traumatizing enough, but in racing around that house, she sprained a leg. Dominos. Sacks of Dread come in a variety of species.

2:Y
10:M
4:D

Surgery completed
February 9 - Journal

Dr. Mahoney completed Drew's cranioplasty today.

Unlike the aborted surgery, Drew seemed tense in the two days before this procedure.

We sat outside the Operating Room (OR) for a couple of hours, snoozed, listened to music and joked. Dr. Mahoney explained the procedure to us, which involved making an incision in his belly from which they removed the fat to inject into his forehead. Seeing an opportunity, I offered my belly fat. He and Drew rejected my offer.

Coming out of surgery Drew only had a couple of small butterfly band-aids on his forehead and some gel in his hair where the incisions had been cut. The suture line was hidden in the hair.

Two hours after he left the OR, I drove us home. We had supper. Amazingly, he stayed up until 11.

During the following 10 days, Drew had some head pain which vanished suddenly. He experienced the worst pain in his stomach, where they removed the fat to inject into his forehead. Every time he turned his body he felt it. Drew regretted that he hadn't taken up my fat offer; I did not.

Drew went back to work after two weeks. He said that he still felt tired and, based on his prior experience, would feel tired for two months.

Just Drew and I went through this surgery; his mother, Rachel, was in Europe with her sister, Marie, at her new home. This is worth mentioning for several reasons. Originally, she had booked her five-week trip to start weeks after the surgery. Then the surgery was delayed—twice. This was not unexpected. If this had been the first surgery, definitely she would have postponed the trip. However, because our new normal included experience with five prior surgeries, four of which were quite serious, and because we knew well the key medical personnel and the procedures, and because Drew was relaxed about the surgery, the rest of us had no qualms about her missing the surgery but she did. However, she knew that it was also very important for her to take a prolonged break. Her sister, who had lived with us at the hospitals from the first hour, would be of tremendous comfort to her.

Therapy dog and I made frequent visits to my mother-in-law at the retirement home, where keeping her unaware of recent events turned out to be a comfort to us more than to her. Even with her deteriorating mental health, her innate powers of observation sharpened by years of nursing told her that something serious was going on that we were keeping from her. Rather than demand details, she had the wisdom to honour our apparent need for secrecy and comforted us instead. Being able to give to us in this way made her feel useful, just like the old times and therefore also benefited her. It's interesting how these things play out.

3 : Y
8 : M

Another sabbatical
December - Journal

In October, Drew began a sabbatical from work, slightly more than 2-years after he returned to work. Drew had gone back to work part-time sixteen months after he was injured. Starting at several half days a week, he worked up to full-time over ten months.

It soon became clear that working, plus commuting 3 hours, exhausted him daily, even more so than it affects all of us and our productivity. But he was determined.

Unfortunately, the company's productivity needs for his marketing position had increased and become more complex. His exhaustion compounded his diminishing, but still present, problems in his still healing brain, negatively affecting his performance. Perhaps more importantly, it also deprived him of energy that his ongoing healing needed, possibly delaying his healing and reducing its quality.

After six months of evaluations and discussions between Drew, his employers and his rehabilitation team it was apparent to all that Drew should take a sabbatical.

You can imagine Drew's stress and mixed emotions during those 6 months. He first heard from the company about their performance review just two days before his brother's wedding. He kept the information to himself so as to not spoil the event. We sensed his stress but did not know the reason. You can see his stress and self-isolation in the wedding photos. As happy as he was for JJ and Alexandra, such an event couldn't help but underscore for him his life situation.

Finally, all agreed that everyone, including Drew, the company and the long-term disability insurer, had rushed Drew's return to work. However, for Drew, it had been imperative that he return to work as soon as possible. As the President of his company explained early on, returning to work was an important incentive milestone for his recovery and self-validation.

Then it got murky. Drew was unclear about what the company proposed. At my suggestion he brought in the law firm that had handled his earlier situation with the insurance company. Their call spooked the company's human resources department until the lawyer explained that it was a call for clarification only since Drew was having difficulties understanding what they were proposing. They hadn't put their proposal in writing, which would have been an appropriate step in dealing with any employee never mind one recovering from a brain injury.

It is possible that even they didn't know exactly what they were required to do and what they were offering, given that their long-term disability insurance company would need to make some decisions about evaluation, compensation and training.

Technically, Drew remains an employee of the company. Whether or not he returns and, if so, to what position is unknown. Approximately 80 percent of people suffering brain injuries do not return to their former jobs as the result of a combination of reduced capacity, setting new life priorities and choosing new, more rewarding occupations.

Since Drew went on sabbatical he has slept 10-11 hours a day. Two months later we noticed that he had become more relaxed, happier, funnier, more insightful, and more playful with Rachel and even with me. It was a wonderful family Christmas present. It is too early to tell if he has any brain performance changes.

As well, with exhaustion absent his gist-reasoning had improved— the ability to create meaning rather than seeing only a collection of unrelated facts. To quote Asha K. Vas MS and Sandra B. Chapman PhD who have studied gist-reasoning in TBI adults, "In essence, gist-reasoning is a perfect example of the adage 'the whole is more than the sum of its parts'."

We don't know when Drew will be ready to move out and back into independent living. No rush; he enriches our lives in many ways. I understand that unmarried brain injured patients often will move out and then return home several times before they are healed enough to deal fully with the demands of independent living. We are doing our best to enable Drew to have the best of both worlds. As housemates, we may be a tad more demanding than most. But then again, Rachel provides Michelin-level-meals and they challenge each other to up their card game skills.

Meanwhile, he and I negotiate the flash points of puns and humour, about which I write below at page 129.

Notes to Nurses, Doctors and Other Health Care Providers

As you know, objectivity, knowledge, expertise, experience, timely data and compassion are critical to your success as a health care professional. Of these, you share only compassion with the patient's family and friends. Even that is inhibited by your necessary professional objectivity and the lack of shared history with the patient.

Even with the obvious distinctions between you, those involved may not recognize all consequences, challenges and opportunities that important distinctions present. I write about them only in this chapter, not in the following chapters, which were written by and for the caregiver who is not a medical professional. Also I recognize the degree to which my observations vary in relevance depending upon the patient's place on the continuum from trauma through acute and critical care to their particular outcome.

The patient's critical needs are obvious, but what about the
condition of the collaterally damaged family and friends? They
aren't furniture. Anticipate their condition and work with it to
achieve multiple positive outcomes. You have the effective hand.

Shock

The close family is in shock; you are not. Throughout their
journey they will experience serial shocks of varying degrees and
the resulting accumulation of adrenalin toxins. We discovered
that when one family member suffers brain injury, all family
members become brain injured. This will both effect and affect
their behaviour. As an example, during Drew's recovery we were
exhibiting *confabulation* too probably due to being forced to figure
out the *new nows* of the moment—Drew's and ours. It was like
being thrown into a version of the game of *Twenty Questions* in
which the first secret to be revealed was that we were playing
Twenty Questions. When we realized that, like Drew, we too were
confabulating we found it funny, in a black humour kind of way.
It was quite common for one of us to say, "Oh, I'm confabulating
again." On reflection, I realize that such group injuries must be
true of the families of all critically injured patients. For you, that
means that you will interact with more patients than just the
official one in the bed.

I suggest to you that recognizing this larger group as patients also
is not a negative. For certain, the patient's friends and family
members can either be a liability or an asset. But by your official
position, your training, your experience, your calling and your
proximity you are in the position to influence, even to determine,
which they are to be. Moreover, I suggest that by handling family
members wisely and skillfully you will turn them into a valuable
asset in your treatment of the critical patient. I suggest also that
by enrolling the patient's family and friends more actively as
caregivers, that you will bring them out of shock and heal these
collaterally damaged. We experienced that benefit.

Power and powerlessness

You have power; the family doesn't. Powerlessness is analogous to coming out of a coma; it is hugely disorienting and frightening. Help them address that feeling of powerlessness using various methods, including some of those suggested below.

Professional knowledge and expertise versus ignorance, superstition and non-medically sanctioned treatments

Your actions, values and world view will be anchored in an evolving *body of knowledge*. Unfortunately, patients and their families behave according to knowledge and world view, values, superstitions and cyberchondria not mediated by that *body of knowledge*. Furthermore, trauma and group dynamics may further distort how they act and believe. Be prepared to modify that behaviour through compassion and education. Keep it simple. Make them part of the health care team as soon as you can in order to avoid the worst manifestations of ignorance, superstition and non-medically sanctioned treatments. Doing so will build active mutual trust at both the interpersonal and professional relationship levels.

Also, doing so will be of help to all concerned if end-of-life discussions become necessary.

Psychological distancing

If you are in ICU or other critical care work, the volume of patients that you see provides you with a necessary psychological distancing mechanism in crises. Otherwise you would have switched into another area of health care.

Family members don't have a choice. However, they can and must build distancing in order to return to health and objectivity. These qualities can evolve to a degree as they see other critically ill patients and meet, befriend and even accompany the families of those patients at the various stages of their respective journeys. Such experience helps them by providing context, relativity, proportionality and perspective. Furthermore, they come to realize that comforting others also helps the comfort-giver, discharging stress being one benefit.

Be prepared for each family that you deal with to change over time. Encourage those changes in positive directions. This will reduce burdens on your time and psyche. Watch for ways that you can influence that process.

Healers

Perhaps you are one of those health care professionals who are healers. I had the honor of knowing, seeing in action and helping set up a cancer research foundation for one such doctor. He also brought out that healing ability in his staff. Some non-health care professionals have comparable gifts. Our ability to explain such a gift is limited. If you have such a gift, appreciate and use it. If you see others with such a gift, health care professionals or family members, use and assist those gifts. You can start that process in a mild way by showing your compassion, showing the family members that you care for their loved one and for them. This will have a beneficial impact on them all, including the patient, and will benefit your working environment.

The risk is that you may be hurt. Find a professional mentor to learn how to strike a balance.

Being useful

Your sense of self-worth will be reinforced by each of the tasks that you do to ensure a positive patient outcome. Initially, families have no such validation. At a time of maximum need they have almost no ability to affect patient outcome, or so they think. Find work for them to do. Make them aware of the very important role they play as part of the health care team. Their resulting improved state of mind will help the patient and make your life a lot easier.

Engage them in doing some of the things that you do as a professional; for example repeatedly asking the patient questions such as *where* and *who* they are, and then affirming correct responses and correcting wrong ones. Make sure that the family understands that in the early stages what is most important is the dialogue, not the accuracy of the patient's answer, which can be sorted out later. Otherwise the family may obsess unnecessarily about the importance of the patient's repeated incorrect answers.

Blood harmony and using the shared past

Patients in comas and patients near death must be helped to orient themselves towards life and the present place and time, which to them are relative to each moment. This realization is very important because we are all on journeys, all of the time. Those asleep, in a coma or trauma are no different in that regard. The difference between them and us is that their grasp of time, spatial orientation, and facts may be completely derailed by their brain injury. They may be unable to tell the difference between reality, dreaming or death. Being unable to tell the difference, in which direction will they orient themselves? My guess is that left alone they will orient themselves towards the near future that they perceive to be the easiest, most pain free or the most peaceful.

I assume, perhaps incorrectly, that our brains strive ceaselessly to make sense of inputs and incorporate them into meaningful directions for its host being—effectively a definition of both movement and of life itself. The opposite is entropy, a state of no energy, which is death.

Although we now know that the brain has great neuroplasticity, we know that neuroplasticity rerewiring is implemented slowly, over considerable time, perhaps as much as 10 years, much like the 10,000 hours required to learn a new skill. However, in order to survive, a traumatized brain needs rewiring immediately. The first 36 hours of healing are the most critical to survival. The brain is drowning in chaos; throw it a rope. To use another drowning metaphor, lifeguards are taught that when rescuing a drowning person they must push the lifejacket or reaching pole firmly, even harshly, into the victim's chest or abdomen. Instinctively, the person at risk will grab it.

You can use your professionalism as that reaching pole; but you do not have with any patient the more effective reaching pole: *blood harmony*. I've borrowed the term *blood harmony* which refers to singing families that are able to achieve magnificent harmonies because of their shared nature and nurture. Unrelated singers, even exceptional ones, can never achieve such harmonies.

A loosely similar medical term is *entrainment*. I urge you to use your professional centrality to this life/death tipping point to immediately engage the family in the many ways that they can use their shared *blood harmony* to guide and to encourage the patient towards life and consciousness. Those many ways include: kissing (olfaction+touch, engaging chemoreceptors); hand holding; massaging; talking; story, joke and news telling; and singing and music playing. See page 103 for specific suggestions for families. Emphasize to the family that until the patient is out of danger they should use these tools as frequently as they can, with the obvious medically necessitated exceptions.

Experience convinced me that this is a powerful tool particularly in the hands of the patient's family and friends and about which they are unlikely to be aware. Now you are. Apply this as a nursing art. Use the family and friends as additional instruments. No training required. Simple, no?

Why you? Well, if not you, who? At such a time, you have three critical things that the family does not have: the objectivity, expertise and experiences in your chosen profession. It is very unlikely that the power of *blood harmony* will occur to the family particularly at the onset of their trauma, at the very time that it is most needed. Direct them, guide them or suggest it to them. If you don't believe in its "unproven" effectiveness, I ask you, "What do you, or most importantly, what does the patient have to lose or to gain by implementing it?" Furthermore, the family and friends are untreated injured. The additional professional benefit that you will create is that by engaging the family in this process, you will heal them by empowering them. By engaging them, they will be relieved to be doing something useful and potentially lifesaving. Furthermore, you reduce their trauma by giving them important tasks, instead of leaving them to flounder in the destructive maelstrom of fear, guilt, helplessness and loss. By consciously using blood harmony, even if their loved one dies, they will live on stronger, knowing that they did their best.

Clearly, your mandated responsibility is to the patient in the bed, not to the collaterally damaged relatives. But you chose your field because of your compassion for *all* people. I suggest that by enlisting that patient's close family and friends effectively in the caregiving process that you will be more effective in treating that patient and will also create the collaterally healed. Even if the patient dies, you will not only take satisfaction in knowing that you did your best for that patient, but you will also take great satisfaction in knowing that you healed many other people walking your community who, in turn, will use their experience to heal others. Call it the power of one—you!

Religious perspectives - the unexplainable

Obviously, religion and cultural experience can be of tremendous help to the patient and the family caregivers. You don't need to have faith, adhere to a religion or even understand why people do. Even if these are placebos, they can be of help and solace. If faith is not a placebo, it can be very powerful. We just don't know; it is destructively arrogant to think otherwise.

As you have read, I experienced the inexplicable with Drew. It was not the result of faith. By nature I am a rationalist; yet I accept what I experienced without either fear or the need to "know". In your career, you may be fortunate enough to have similar inexplicable experiences.

Shifts away

When *you* leave the hospital, quite properly and necessarily you leave the trauma behind. The family can't and don't. In the family, the toxins build and their energy diminishes. This has negative consequences. Encourage the family to take days off. They need that survival instinct validated and guilt removed by an experienced professional whom they trust. ICU staff wisely counselled us to take breaks, even while Drew was still in ICU and, therefore, still critical. Don't assume that your more experienced colleagues on the team have advised the family to take breaks. In any case, in this situation repeating such advice is likely to be required before it registers with those in shock.

Even if you are not in critical-care but subsequently treat former critical-care patients and their families, you have a role to play in this regard. Safely away from the traumatic crisis and further along the road to recovery, recommend to both patient and families that they consider taking an extended, restorative break, even allowing themselves to descend into zero-pulse days. By doing so, they will gain perspective and energy and therefore be better able to continue the recovery.

Note that I mentioned giving such advice to the patient as well. For reasons concerning fear, confusion, self-validation and personal drive, patients can attempt to force improvements that only time can provide. Premature, counterproductive and even dangerous examples include the patient's too early eagerness to travel independently, take over their financial affairs, return to work and live independently. Explain to both patient and family why they must be cautious. It is best for all concerned if the patient *facilitates* healing and does not fallaciously attempt to *control* healing. We always referred to Drew's healing as his sabbatical; it was important but temporary.

Humour

I understand that the areas of the brain devoted to crying and laughing are co-located. Black humour will surface and may not be appreciated by some family members but it is a useful means of releasing stress and orienting patient and family to the good times, as well as putting the bad times to rest.

Two months after Drew's injury, his last night in the third hospital, Drew, JJ and I were sitting at a picnic table outside the hospital on a beautiful June evening enjoying Tim Hortons' Danishes and coffee.

Drew mentioned that some visitors to the hospital had asked him if he was really a patient. Uninhibitedly he replied to them, "I was hit by a train." Then he took his knitted cap off, which he also did while telling us the story. This revealed his skull-absent, sloping, scarred, misshapen forehead, and the scar line over the top of his head from ear to ear. Then he said to these people, "What do you think?"

The effect was so startling, even to JJ and me, that all three of us broke out into raucous, tear-inducing, stomach-aching laughter.

"I did get a sense of how shocking it is to people," Drew said, precipitating us into another fit of laughter.

I guess you had to be there. But, those poor unsuspecting people… Be prepared for your own such moments. They are cathartic.

Thank you

You will be thanked many times in your career, but it will never be enough. However, I suggest that you won't be short-changed; by giving, you will receive manifold. There are many belief systems that have this as a central tenet. I believe that psychologists have evidence proving that you receive psychological benefits when you give. We wish for you that every day you are able to take a few moments to reflect on your day's giving, so as to receive and to allow yourself to experience those daily blessings. You earn them.

And now, back to our journey with Drew, other patients, and their families and friends.

The Hospital System – Our Experience

As might be expected given Drew's miraculous progress, we are very positive about the quality of care that Drew received from the police, Emergency Medical Services (EMS) and the staff of the four hospitals. I hope your experience is just as positive and I will suggest ways for you to make it the best that you can.

First, remember that the health care professionals are responsible to the patient not to you. They interact with you in order to treat the patient, even though you may have some temporary form of legal guardianship of the patient. If there is a conflict about treatment between what you—the non-medical family member—want and what the medical experts believe is the best course of action for the patient, they will side with the patient. That is the way it should be. If you were the patient it is what you would want. Bearing this in mind, you can still be a valuable, influential member of the health care team.

It is important to remember always that the NeuroTrauma ICU medical and other staff have dedicated their lives to helping patients like your loved one. They are highly trained and committed. Their job is in a very high demand, high stress environment. They must avoid becoming caught up in your emotions in order to do their job to the best of their training, talents and skills. Therefore, don't ever take their professionalism as a sign that they don't care about you and your loved one.

The staff knows that you are beyond stressed, in a place with no rational or even emotional norms, with no shared experience, language or descriptive terms for your condition. They know that what you are going through is totally experiential and that no analysis or understanding of it is possible nor can it be communicated. They know that now you communicate as if you are learning to speak a second language. They know the stakes. Some are better at it than others. Some days they are better at it than on others, due to experience, training, personality and how their day has gone.

But know this: whether or not your loved one receives exceptional care beyond high quality care depends greatly upon you—the family members. You are the patient's primary advocate and caregiver.

All of the following can play a significant part in whether or not you ensure an exceptional level of quality of care. Essentially, these observations fall into two categories: state of mind; and, actions. Both apply to you and to the professionals. Even within their objective professionalism, the staff will respond positively to the following.

Your loved one is a person

Perhaps the single most important thing you can do is to help the medical staff get to know your loved one as a wonderful person in your life. Establish your loved one as a human being with a personality and a life, rather than as meat on a bed—a case. All of us go the extra mile for someone we know and like.

At all times introduce them to each other by name, for example: "Drew, Dr. Singh is here". Also, it is far more than a phrase to say "bring your loved one to life" by putting up photos of your loved one, not portraits but candid photos of them living their life and photos of them in situations with the hospital-visiting family and friends, so that staff see the family resemblances and make the connections. If the photo shows that the patient looks like you, then each time you speak with the nurses or Doctors you will bring the patient to life for them. It is your behaviour that presents the patient as a wonderful human being or an out-of-control jerk.

Play the loved one's favourite music or recorded voice messages from friends and family. Such measures will bring life orientation to your caregiving and patient-advocacy roles, and everyone, including medical staff and your family, will respond positively. So will your loved one.

Treating them normally will trigger memories, even in their coma and their injured brain, which will help them orient themselves and their will, in the direction of life.

Courtesy, respect and warmth

Treat all medical professionals with courtesy, respect and warmth. If they like you, by extension they will be inclined to like the patient too.

As best you can, keep your emotions under control. Never insult or attack staff no matter how right you think you are. If you do "lose it", apologize immediately or have a family member apologize on your behalf.

Consult a hospital social worker if you think that you aren't being heard by medical staff or need help.

Thank you motivates – good manners with a purpose

Warmly thank staff regularly, even daily, for helping your loved one. Bring cookies and brownies to the nursing station. Home-made, even friend-made baking is a great motivator of staff—they will know that they are enjoying what your loved one has also enjoyed.

Thanking staff, family, and friends will focus you on the positive and it will boost your morale.

Track treatment details in a Log or Journal and speak up

Create a patient log or journal. Monitor and write down in the log all test results, electronic monitor status changes and treatments, medications, the name of the treating health care professional and the time of day of these events.

Make certain that an informed family member is present in NeuroTrauma ICU for at least one of the daily doctors' rounds, which are usually twice a day, and listen in on what the doctors and nurses are discussing. Ask questions politely and speak up if something doesn't sound right, such as the doctor ordering a new course of antibiotics to which you know that the patient is allergic—Rachel did. They will get used to you being there and eventually will come to trust you and even include you in the discussions as they did with Rachel.

You may think that this activity is pointless and perhaps even worse because you are an amateur attempting to second-guess the professionals. Also, you may think that such participation is overly cautious belts-and-suspenders at best. Even amateurs can record data and report observations; understanding it is something else. You will come to learn and understand more and more. Astute observations can be helpful to the professional team. You and the professional medical team have a single objective: a positive patient outcome. If by your data and your questions you bring to light a dangerous anomaly, they will thank you. If you ask a reasonable question, they will explain. They know that you are part of the health care team too and that you could make a significant contribution.

Moreover, this activity focuses your energy in positive directions, and it increases your knowledge which makes you a better advocate and caregiver. Undertaking this vital activity will give you additional important benefits such as giving you something to do during long hours of boredom so that stress and fears don't have time to consume you.

Combined, these activities will improve the quality of the care for your loved one and their outcome.

The mirror test

At the start of each day, look at yourself in the mirror. Do you think positively of the person that you see there? Would your loved one like to see you looking like this? Yes you will see the ravages of stress there; it is what it is.

However, both men and women can and need to be well dressed and groomed as if you are going to an important meeting and want to make a good impression—you are, you do, you must.

This may seem to be a ridiculously trivial or superficial point at a time when your concern should be for your seriously injured loved one. It is neither trivial nor superficial.

The daily self-disciplining *ritual act* of dressing and grooming will provide you with a controllable routine at the beginning of each day in order to put on your *game face*. The ritual will be a time of reflection that you must use to focus on both the longer term and that day's objectives. If you don't put yourself through that ritual daily, you will probably lapse into obsessing about stepping back into chaos. Such thoughts will rupture your Sack of Dread and you will feel and look worse than awful. Certainly you will be in no condition to drive a car safely.

On the other hand, putting yourself through this grooming ritual will calm you down. Together, calmness, grooming and dressing well will achieve a number of important objectives.

Your calmer appearance will calm your family and visitors. By presenting itself well, the family will signal to the health care professionals that its members and your injured loved one should be treated extra seriously and with extra respect, compassion and effort. Remember that people make these judgments subconsciously—at an animal or Darwinian level.

If you doubt this, look at yourself in the mirror again. Positive or negative? If that is what you think, then why would others think any differently? If the mirror confirms that this happens to be one of the days when you are *losing it*, seriously consider staying away, taking a break and arranging for others to fulfill your responsibilities. That judgment would be in your loved one's best interest and yours too.

The health care professionals should take you as you are? Remember, any impression that you give reflects upon the patient. If you aren't willing to do your best for your loved one, then stay away. This is not about you.

Rules

Follow hospital rules as best you can. They are there for a reason even if you don't understand the reason. If you need to know it, ask. Don't risk creating conflict that may create more stress.

Examples of such rules are:

- Visiting hours – These are somewhat flexible for immediate next-of-kin such as parents, adult children, and spouses and can be discussed with ward staff

- Number of simultaneous visitors allowed

- Where you can and cannot use mobile phones and computers or smoke

- Sanitizing your hands entering and leaving the hospital, the floor, the ward and before and after touching the patient

- Don't disrupt the patient. Stay away if you might disrupt because you may be ill, weak or distraught

- Find out what are banned items, such as flowers, and don't bring them

- Inform your expected visitors about the rules **before** they arrive. Spread the word through your new social media site.

Your Caregiver Team

While this part is written primarily for close family members, it can also assist the health care professional who deals with them. The following individual items will have differing degrees of relevance to various stages of the journey. For the most part, they are weighted towards the critical care stage. There are two focused sections: on page 107, Critical Care, and on page 110, Non-Critical Care. Think of the following as a reference list with explanations. In the appendices, you will find several To Do Handout lists to which you can refer Family and Friends in order to assist them organize the extended caregiver community.

It is important to describe the role that my wife, Rachel, played and plays today in giving care to our son Drew. I don't know where she found the strength but I do know where she found the ability. As a role model, she had her mother, a former take-charge nurse. Also, raising three sons gives mothers something of an undergraduate degree in medicine.

Over the 18-months prior to Drew's injury, Rachel and her sister Marie gained many exhausting months of experience with health care. In a city a two-hour drive away, they cared for their then 90-year-old mother as she underwent hip surgery and related traumas necessitating extended hospital care; temporary long-term care; exchanging her apartment for a retirement home; and then changing cities for a different long-term care facility. This was on top of Rachel's own energy-sapping health challenges.

I mention Rachel's story both because it is extraordinary and it highlights the fact that we all arrive in a crisis with different strengths and weaknesses. Looking at Rachel as an *everyperson*, we can draw two important conclusions. First, all of us can rise to the challenge, overcoming a wide variety of shortcomings and drawing on strengths that we didn't know we had. Second, we—you—all have different assets to contribute to the well-being of the patient and to the team.

Early on, inventory the team's known strengths and weaknesses. Don't be surprised if, with encouragement, team members excel in ways that you could not have imagined. As another team member, thank them for shouldering part of the load so very well. Surprisingly, many people do not recognize the value of something exceptional that they do, or skills or talents that they have. Giving such recognition will strengthen the team and the individuals on it.

You as motivator, you as guide

Caregiver is easy to understand; but *motivator* and *guide*?

Based on our caregiver team's experience we learned there are quite a few things you can do that will help your loved one and improve your time as a caregiver. To simplify presentation they are recommended to you as lessons we learned that you can modify to your circumstances and implement as appropriate.

You are critical and essential to your loved one's survival in ways that the medical staff, even as wonderful and experienced as they may be, cannot possibly duplicate. It is up to you to ensure that the patient maintains the will to survive and to heal. To do so, you must be a familiar, comforting, encouraging and constant presence penetrating their pain and mental chaos.

You must constantly, constantly make your loved one aware of you. They must constantly know that you are accompanying them on their path to recovery. A very appropriate analogy is that of a parent coaxing their infant through its first steps—from an arm's length ahead—perhaps letting them grasp your finger for a sense of security. Tears are common at such times, for many reasons. Don't be afraid to let them flow when you are celebrating improvement.

Accompanying the patient is an active not a passive role. Just being in the same room with them is not enough.

While their mind and body may have an instinct to survive, they may not have a will to survive. In my experience, they are not at all the same. Do I have proof? No. But it was obvious that there was no downside to acting and there were many probable upsides. Do I have anecdotal corroboration from others? Yes. Recently, a good friend described a similar *presence-experience* that she had with her father when he was near death after a major stroke, which he then survived. Also, I understand that there are many similar reports available. There are certainly many bright-light reports from survivors of death or near death experiences. Force yourself between your loved one and that seductive light. Make your loved one make you their destination instead.

A month into our journey, I met a patient who had already spent a year in NeuroTrauma ICU in varying degrees of a coma-like paralysis suffering from Guillain–Barré Syndrome. He said that even in total paralysis he heard everything. Visitors didn't censure themselves, saying things that were highly distressing to him because they took his lack of responsiveness to mean that he could hear nothing. The offenders included medical staff, relatives and friends. Occasionally these remarks made him suicidal. "Fortunately," he said, "I could not act on those feelings but I did think about stopping fighting to live." He could not do *anything*. But, he had the power to do *nothing*.

My final example is Dr. Jill Bolte Taylor, a neuroanatomist, who had a major stroke, survived it and after years of recovery now writes and talks about it from the inside. She has spoken to the TED Conference and on Oprah Winfrey, both of which can be found on line and on YouTube. Her book, My *Stroke of Insight*, is a tremendous resource book for patients and caregivers alike. In it she describes a more worrisome patient condition, that is, not wanting to come back from the wonderful mystical state that she found herself in, where there was no boundary between her body and the world. She experienced herself at the molecular level that was at one with the universe. When she gives talks she tries to persuade people to put themselves in that state of awareness in order to make a better world.

If the severely injured is more comfortable *out of their body*, will they want to stay there? If the visitors to their hospital room reflect to the patient a chaotic, fragmented existence of pain, anguish, and negativity would they want to go **there**? Would you? "Perhaps" is not an acceptable answer.

Even before learning of these examples, I knew that there was too much risk in doing nothing and no risk at all in doing everything. My first bedside experience with Drew absolutely convinced me. I had no knowledge of what I was dealing with but sensed that I was dealing with Drew's essence and, simultaneously, separately with his body, his senses and his brain. I sensed that for him to live that he needed to unite these necessary elements of himself. I felt that it was extremely important that all of us orient Drew to life at all times, that we make life highly desirable and that we continually guide him towards it.

His survival can't be taken as proof; but, hey, it works for me.

Earthquake struck warehouse

Think of it this way. The injured brain is like a warehouse hit by an earthquake that throws shelves and inventory into a jumble on the floor. The injured brain has to pick up each piece and place it on the correct shelf. How can they do that when they don't know what shelves are or what each object is or why they should straighten up the chaos? Imagine being them, in a world that is without up or down, past, present or future. They are unable to distinguish between the equally attractive memory, dream or afterlife. They have no reason to focus on one over the other. Where do they start?

They are at an unidentifiable intersection between infinity and eternity. They are in a completely disoriented world and need focus and direction. Having neither orientation nor direction, how do they move towards life and health? You.

They are a chaos of perceptions without knowledge of what or who they are—without meaning. In that state it is up to you to make them recognize what and who **you** are. The rest will follow.

First of all, they must relate to you.

Applying *blood harmony*

As mentioned previously, the term *blood harmony* refers to singing families that are able to achieve magnificent harmonies because of their shared nature and nurture. Even exceptional but unrelated singers can never achieve such harmonies. The same connectedness occurs in other aspects of family life.

Applying *blood harmony*, you make the patient relate to you through their senses which can continue to function even when they are in a coma. Deep in their DNA and in their memory are both your patterns and their patterns of their relationship with you—blood harmony. These are rich, detailed, complex resources for you both. Forcing them to engage with those resources, will re-establish both their sense of self and a direction—the linkage with you. Most importantly, this makes them aware that they are still alive, which is critical to them finding the will to live. Then they can begin to move towards you, towards life.

Importantly, *blood harmony* is that supremely powerful tool which family members have which medical professionals do *not* have. There is more on the subject at page 87.

To unlock this life saving power, immediately and continuously you must play both their senses and their sensory memory like a musical instrument.

Of the tactile input options, kissing may sound frivolous but your kiss is unique with respect to touch (pressure, duration, skin to skin engagement) and your unique odours both natural and cosmetic. Odours feed the powerful sense of smell which in turn sequentially stimulates many parts of the brain. According to Sheril Kirshenbaum, biologist and author of *The Science of Kissing* "Our sense of smell tells us a lot about other people .... It happens on a subconscious level and kissing puts us in the closest proximity possible to get a sample. Women have a stronger sense of smell and taste and when we are kissing we use the information we get from our senses. It is nature's ultimate litmus test".

You have kissed them, now they know *who* you are but they don't necessarily know *when* you are. You still need to help the patient distinguish the present-you from the past-you. The moment-to-moment present is uncertain and therefore, by our evolved survival nature, demands great concentration. Memories, on the other hand, have relivable, predictable story lines which the patient may find less demanding. Families, friends and health care professionals must be more demanding, thereby orienting the patient to the present and to the future, to the living, therefore to life.

Again, this is a critical area where families and close friends have the knowledge, and embedded links with the patient that no health care professional can access. Use all the many tactile inputs, in addition to kissing: hand holding; massaging; talking; story, joke and news telling; and singing and music playing.

Reinforce your link every time you enter or leave their presence, by greeting the patient or saying good-bye—using your and their name. Tell them that you are going to the washroom, making a phone call, meeting with the therapist or going to get some coffee, and tell them that you will be back shortly. It helps them re-establish the concept of present and future and reassures them, even though specific time and even relative time may have little or no meaning.

Imitate the professionals – "Where are you?"

Find out from the doctors and nurses what they are doing to test the comatose patient's change in neural function and to orient them. The staff will pinch patients or induce pain by pushing a knuckle into the breast bone to provoke a pain response which tells them about the patient's state of neural functioning. At different stages there will be different neural functioning and different states of sensory awareness about which you may not know. When the patient is out of the coma, every few minutes staff will ask them where they are, get them to repeat it and correct wrong answers. You do the same. Leave the knuckle test to the professionals.

Read and re-read to them

Since you must assume that they can hear you, talk to them all the time. Read and re-read notes from well-wishers. Read the newspaper or their favourite magazines or books. Tell them gossip, sports scores, the news and jokes. All of these things connect them to the world they knew and, given choice, motivation and direction, will want to rejoin.

No negative talk

Establish a calm normal. Don't say anything negative near them and only talk about them out of earshot, even with doctors, nurses or caregivers. Discussing simple things with the nurses or doctors is fine.

If you need to cry, and you will, leave the bedside. They don't need either the stress or more motivation to give up hope and then stop fighting for life and healing.

Inform yourself

Inform yourself as best you can about the patient's condition. Read the hospital literature and share it with others on your family caregiver team. Knowledge reduces fear and stress. The material gives you signs of progress to look for and provides a realistic, but not exact, time frame. Print it out and use it to fill in time while at the bed side or taking a break in the cafeteria. If there are things that you don't understand, ask the nurses, doctors, therapists or social workers.

Bizarre behaviour

Watch for repeated bizarre phrases or behaviour and try to understand what the patient thinks they are saying or doing. The patient will assume that they are being *normal*. To the rest of us they are just being weird, or even dangerous to themselves. You will share a huge inventory of pre-injury experiences with the patient that may help to unlock some of these mysteries. Out of earshot of the patient, your family caregiving team can speculate and work together to find an explanation. Think of it as *Charades* or *Twenty Questions*. Unexpected humour, some of it black, will surface at such times. Let it flow. Participate. Not only will it reduce stress but it will build a stronger team and, therefore, will find faster the explanation of the bizarre.

An example of this is when repeatedly Drew took off the cervical collar which was around his neck to allow a fractured neck vertebrae to heal. No doubt, the collar was both unfamiliar and uncomfortable. But removing the collar put him in danger of paralysis.

This behaviour started almost as soon as he was out of wrist restraints and was able to sit up unsupported. It went on for at least a month. It became even more bizarre when he started removing the collar from his neck and placing it on top of his head.

Driving home one night, wondering why he was doing it, an idea came to me out of the blue. On my next visit, when he put the collar on his head, I said to him, "Drew, you are not DJing a club. That collar around your neck is not a headset. It's a neck brace to protect you. Leave it on." From that day on, Drew took it off only for a good reason. Drew had been a musician for many years and in recent years had been DJing events. DJs need to use a headset and often place it across the top of their heads so that only one ear piece is in use, leaving the other ear to hear the music in the room.

So you now see that it was rational—to Drew. But, initially, it wasn't rational within our frame of reference. Remember that reality of differing world views. Keeping it front of mind will help you during the many, many differences and conflicts that you will have with the patient.

It might also help you to think of the patient's reality as your very own, interactive, serialized graphic novel.

Critical Care - the routine practicalities

Find the time and energy to help others who might be your loved one's partners, close friends, co-workers, or roommates. You may be surprised at the benefits you receive. These people will be distressed and feeling helpless. Depending upon the cause of the trauma, they may even feel guilty and concerned that in some way you, the family, also hold them accountable or partially to blame. It is not reasonable to think this way, but this is not a reasonable time. Let them know that you care for them as important people in your loved one's life.

Only as I finished this book did I become conscious of two other very important players inside our new now—Drew the *person-in-and-of-the world* and the representative of him in that world, Maria, for want of a better term, his *angel*.

Neil and Maria had been in contact almost immediately. She had been close to Drew. They had been together a few days before his accident. Apparently, she wanted to visit Drew in the hospital, which I said would not be possible. We knew very little about her. I had met her only once when she dropped by with Drew to pick up some camping gear on their way to join several hundred of their friends who got together often, including canoeing into the bush to camp, play music and socialise on long weekends. Since I suspected that she might be feeling distraught and perhaps even guilty, I agreed that Neil should arrange for the 3 of us to meet.

At that meeting she was very striking—calm and very centred. It turned out—to my surprise—that she was a lawyer. I agreed that Neil would arrange for her visits to Drew—only when Rachel and I were absent.

Families can wallow in their grief; they can be rudderless. I now believe that Maria added an important dimension to our perception of the Drew we were fighting for, a reinforcing external validation of our fight—not that we needed it. This Drew was larger, and more multi-faceted, more interconnected with and important to the world. Our lives in the world are seldom tangible to our families. We knew that Drew was more than son and brother but we had little appreciation of how important he was in the lives of others. Naturally, his brothers had experienced more of this than his parents.

Maria visited Drew daily—frequently twice daily. One evening, by accident she was there when Rachel and I arrived. Arriving from her law office, she was imposing in her stylish suit, well groomed and made-up. She smiled warmly, entering our hearts. From then on she came and went with our blessing. She represented to us— and to hospital staff, patients and visitors—that powerful other dimension of Drew about which we had only vaguely been aware.

At the time we were so focused that I was only slightly aware of a most important additional dimension of Maria's impact on Drew's recovery. She was able to trigger his memories and to remind him of who he was and of the nature of his relationships with other people in his life. It was important for him to have more than just family with him during recovery and to know that he was and is loved by many people. Due to her prior relationship with him and her intelligence, sensitivity, compassion and love she proved to be an exceptional representative of the best qualities of Drew's remarkable community of friends—as I was to discover in the weeks and months ahead.

Also, because of her prior relationship with Drew she knew that she could be an important non-family sounding board, freeing him to express what he was thinking and feeling and to give him reasonable feedback on both. Even in his severely injured vulnerability and self-doubt, he was able to compare and contrast two sets of reactions and advice thereby enabling him to arrive at understanding on which he could then act. He valued the inputs of both groups but—quite rightly—he knew that his family's reactions and advice might be influenced by stress or typical family dynamics. Due to their prior close experience, as she had foreseen he trusted and respected Maria to give him objective feedback. We trusted Maria with Drew too. Not only did she radiate trustworthiness, but we knew that in addition to her relationship with Drew, she was trained and experienced in being objective in stressful situations and in advising stressed clients—even though her experience was as a litigator, a courtroom lawyer.

We—particularly Drew—were fortunate that Maria *made* herself that presence, and that is the only way I can put it. Be aware that, as well as you may be coping, it is impossible to be all-seeing, all-knowing and all-wise. Keep yourself open to the Marias, the angels, who materialize at the time of your greatest need and bring important unforeseen gifts. In spite of your Sacks of Dread be open to those possibilities. If you are not receptive, you may not be fortunate enough to have someone as determined as Maria was.

There were many others who, over time, conveyed to us various aspects of Drew's larger importance in the world. One friend made an appointment with Drew to visit him in the hospital. On the way to that appointment on his motorcycle, he injured himself in an accident and yet, even though he was late, he still kept the appointment that he knew was important to Drew as well as to himself. But, for Drew more so than for us, Maria became the daily presence reminding him of his world. In a positive sense I began to take Maria's presence for granted. Then one afternoon—as I silently entered Drew's room where Maria was sitting at the end of the bed—I saw on her unguarded face the love and the pain. That profoundly moving experience had a great impact on me. Such moments, such revelations will visit you.

Non-Critical Care - the routine practicalities

Once in a ward or on the floor or at home, your loved one will depend a great deal more on your non-health care professional caregiving-team for two reasons: first, the constantly hovering health care professional team will no longer be there since the patient no longer needs survival attention; second, the patient will become more demanding and there will be much that they can't do for themselves and fewer professional resources to assist them. By the way, your community-centric caregiver team may not be health care professionals but they may be very experienced caregivers. Think of them that way and treat them accordingly, with frequent evidence of your gratitude.

There are quite a few things that you can do that will help your loved one. The doctors and therapists will provide guidance, direction and exercises. For example, Rachel and Drew would take walks several times a day. In the beginning they were slow, slow, slow. The walks were important in order to restore balance, and rebuild bone and extensive muscle mass lost while in bed. During the walks they would play word games suggested by the therapists to enhance cognitive rehabilitation. In the beginning the games were as simple as naming as many animals as possible that started with each letter of the alphabet. They played the same games for months. Soon they added card games, the playing of which so enhanced both their skills that they often clean-up during family tournaments.

One or more of you will spend much time dealing with bureaucracies and paperwork and the forgetful patient. Let's hear it for Rachel! You will also spend a great deal of time driving your loved one to therapy and other appointments. You will sit in on many meetings and accompany the patient. Accompanying is a special role, like being an interpreter. It is both necessary and a privilege.

In the beginning, the patient is no longer practically nor legally competent to be in charge of themselves. As they recover by degrees, their practical and legal responsibility for themselves will change by degrees too. As the patient is increasingly able to interact intelligently and responsibly on their own behalf, the health care professionals and the institutions will, appropriately, treat you differently, effectively diminishing your role. At a certain point in recovery, you are no longer legally required. This disengagement is a delicate and variable process that, to be done effectively in the best interest of the patient, requires the intelligence, objectivity, judgment, respect and basic humanity of all three parties. Anticipate it and prepare yourself and the patient accordingly.

Your ongoing accompaniment of the patient requires the patient's trust and explicit permission from the patient and their doctors, therapists, employers and insurance companies. You accompany the patient by their permission. You have no power but you have influence, which you relinquish gradually over time. If you behave, you will be seen by all to be a mentor to the patient, a wise friend, an honoured role probably for life. For all concerned you must be wise, patient, forbearing and subtle when you contribute. If you are not, you will be counterproductive, damaging to the patient and will be excluded.

You are not expected to be perfect but you must recognize your imperfections and you must consciously and visibly allow others to see your effort as a work-in-progress, as is the patient. If you do so, your loved one will allow you to see their vulnerability in all of their self-doubt and confusion. This is a rare privilege few of us allow any other. This gives you tremendous power, and therefore tremendous responsibility. Treat your loved one with all the love, respect and nurturing of which you are capable.

Even as the patient is a new window into the world for you, so accompanying the patient will also enrich your life in pleasant, unforeseen ways. For example, having delivered your loved one to their regular therapy or appointments, you will talk with other patients or staff, find shady, inexpensive places to park nearby. You will walk therapy dog, reflect, read, make business calls, think or snooze. You will have hours at a time to explore nearby parts of the city. You will use the time to shop or lunch nearby with old friends.

Over these journeys you will spend much time with your loved one, have many discussions and build many cherished memories. You will come to appreciate them and by extension, others, for what they are, rather than judge them for what they are not.

Patient's employer

Regularly update the most senior person you can reach in the patient's employer firm. Thank them for their support, particularly if you are uncertain about the degree of support that they may be providing. Even consider sending a letter to the president of the company. It would not be inappropriate and could be very helpful over the following months and years. Your patient needs their sympathy and ongoing support for many months; you don't want the patient to fade from awareness and be *downsized*. Drew's firm was great from day one, from the president on down.

Give your lawyer's name and contact information to your loved one's employer. They need to know who to deal with. Furthermore, by doing so you will send them important signals as well. Few employers deal with their employees with the humanism and professionalism that Drew's employer has dealt with him.

Because Drew's company treated Drew so well, we did not involve a lawyer in dealings with them until a second sabbatical was required. At that point Drew was not able to clearly understand the discussions he was having with his company's Human Resources department, a state that even many healthy employees find themselves in too. I recommended to Drew that he have his insurance lawyer, who also had expertise with employment law, call the company to clarify things. Initially the HR department was alarmed at this development but Drew's lawyer calmed them down and within minutes they sorted out the situation satisfactorily for all concerned.

Insurers

Deal appropriately with the insurers from day one. Since the insurer may be the only mechanism able to provide your loved one with necessary financial support for life. *Appropriately* means that it is imperative that you engage a lawyer with insurance company expertise to deal with the insurer from the **first** phone call. It is essential that whoever deals with the insurer on behalf of the patient understands the insurer's protocols and priorities, insurance jurisprudence, and insurer language. If your lawyer has experience with the insurer in question, then so much the better. You don't have either the expertise or the state of mind to deal with the insurer appropriately in the beginning.

The call from a lawyer to the insurer will galvanize the insurer's claims department into action and more quickly bump the patient's claim up the chain of command to a decision-maker in the insurance company. Immediately they will know that you will do whatever is necessary to protect your loved one.

You may think you can save money by dealing with the insurer yourself instead of engaging a lawyer. Wrong. Not using a lawyer in the beginning will cost you and your loved one much more. The initial legal fees will be a reasonable, small investment in order to achieve financial security and remove worries for all concerned. This is particularly important for patients who will not return to work because at the two-year mark the insurer may decide to write a large cheque to cover lifetime support. Engaging a lawyer to represent the patient from the beginning will tip the company closer to a timely fair settlement and away from the expense of litigation and a court ordered settlement.

At the appropriate time someone in your family, properly counselled by your lawyer, can take over the routine reporting as well as making certain that doctors complete necessary medical paperwork which either they or you will file with the insurer. This important task requires much effort, attention to deadlines and details, and many phone calls. Eventually, with coaching, the patient may be able to handle some of this but will need to be monitored to make certain that no mistakes are made or deadlines missed. Remember that brain injuries present additional risks in that regard. Accompany them on all meetings and phone calls until they are absolutely out of danger from the insurer.

I don't wish to leave the impression that either the insurers or employers are villians. Unfortunately, you have to assume that the primary responsibility of the staff of both companies is to their company—not to your loved one. Insurers deal with a great many fraudulent claims; consequently the onus is on you to prove your claim. Unfortunately, in proving your claim, without the assistance of insurance experts who are responsible only to the patient, you and your loved one can innocently make mistakes or use terminology incorrectly or do something else that places the insurance claim in jeopardy. Don't risk it. Engage competent help.

Men and Fathers — Joining the OAJS

At noon of the day following JJ and Alexandra's wedding, very close friends who had attended the wedding called to say that the Montreal police had just told them that their twenty-three year old son, Rick, watching the sunrise with friends after an all-night party had slipped and fallen four stories off a roof and was in NeuroTrauma ICU.

They had followed our 3-year journey with Drew closely, reading Facebook daily and many months later talking in person. At the wedding the day before, Drew told them about how important music and voices had been to guide him out of his coma. Now they called us frequently from the Montreal hospital with many questions and much anguish. Then their son began to show probable signs of surviving. Then he showed signs of probable lack of paralysis. Then after vertebrae fusing, wiring shut his badly fractured jaw and other surgeries, he began a rapid recovery. During his recovery he passed through some very difficult stages, including lack of inhibition and aggression.

These calls were difficult for me. During one of them I listened to the father's outburst. It was a cocktail of relief, frustration and anger. When he had vented, I replied in a spontaneous manner appropriate to our relationship and to our shared experience. "I will need to check with the other members, but I think that you now qualify for admission to the OAJS, the Order of the Asbestos

Jock Strap." Our shared laughter temporarily dissipated much of our trial-by-fire stress. I emailed him a portion of an early draft of this text, which he found helpful.

Miraculously, Rick survived and returned to university six months later, and as he told me during a visit, with the perfect posture that he had always wanted. Two months after his wholly understandable but premature return to university, his body and mind rebelled. Neither one was yet healed enough to accommodate the demands placed on them. Now, with the help of professionals, he is learning to better manage his recovery, a need common to all such patients—and their families.

During a summer's visit to us with his parents, he showed me with pride the precise, 18-inch surgeon's scar down his spine where they fused his vertebrae. Paired on each side of the scar were many puncture scars from the staples used to close up the incision, perfectly spaced about 3/8ths of an inch apart, one above another. He considered adding a pull-tab tattooed at the top of his "zipper" body piercings. Yes, he and Drew have also qualified to join the Order. In case you haven't already guessed, it's a guy thing.

Originally, when psychotherapist Ramona Bray asked me to write a piece for her acquired brain injury Resource Manual, she gave me, as a representative male and father, four questions which I answer below in five words or less and then move on to address them all together.

- The nature/societal challenge - expressing emotion?

- Do fathers have more pressure to comfort and take charge of the existing family and manage their own shock, grief? *No*

- Should fathers behave differently than mothers? *Yes and no*

- Do fathers have a different experience than mothers, siblings, friends? *A qualified yes and no*

For the most part, the To Do lists are handled elsewhere in this book, including the handout lists in the Appendices. Therefore, this part will address the male context and exceptions, starting with the elephant in the room—destructive emotions. It will also deal separately with stress. For the most part I treat stress as the buildup of negative psychological and physiological forces and I treat emotions as the out-of-control volcanic eruption of these massive negative forces. I ignore minor emotional displays.

Fight, flight or freeze

Traumatic events trigger instincts: fight, flight or freeze. Each of us reacts to emergencies differently. I suspect that evolutionary forces have DNA-wired men predisposed to the first two.

Emotions cannot be avoided. However, extreme emotions taking control at the wrong times will harm the patient because they prevent the caregivers from thinking clearly and acting effectively.

There are three time periods for which different responses are appropriate. Assuming that you were not present for the initial trauma, to start there is little that you can do except get to the hospital. Once there you will learn details of the patient's condition but there is little that you can do to help the patient who is in the hands of the health professionals. It is completely appropriate to be emotional at that time and to let off some of the pressure. I would suggest that after half an hour or so, it is time to move to phase two—to suppress the emotions in order to be able to plan schedules and concrete tasks and to divide up responsibilities. That phase can last for months and will be punctuated by emotional explosions. The third phase occurs sometime after you no longer need to hold it together. Then something unforeseen will trigger a meltdown, as I described above at page 51 and below at page 119. That meltdown may last some time and need medication and counselling. Mine did.

Some men and some women excel in dealing with traumatic events due to their DNA and life experience. In no way is that observation a judgment about the value of those who *can't* cope with such traumas. Their gifts may become important later. Those who were excellent in the emergency may be of less value in the days, months and years to come. They may crash then as their suppressed stress and emotions surface. Or, they may have become adrenalin junkies. They may feel impotent, frustrated, or angry.

I now believe that, by removing any realistic hope, the first surgeon actually helped us. I will never know for certain, but if he had not removed all hope I probably would not have had that extraordinary first bedside experience with Drew, that I described above at Sitting With Drew (page 24) and not having had it, Drew may not be alive today.

At such times, behaving inappropriately or emotionally according to artificial, harmful standards imposed by yourself, your family, or your culture is destructive and wrong. For example, establishing caregiver responsibilities according to some abstract cultural norm, such as male absolutism, guarantees additional risk for the patient and psychological and social harm to the caregivers. Judge what you should do according to what the patient and the vulnerable need. There is no other standard.

Emotions: Immediate/Subsequent Experience/Discuss

Everyone's emotional state will change over the hours, days, weeks, months and years following the bomb-blast that resets everyone's emotions. Most aspects of emotions are common to all, regardless of sex, even though they may differ in colour and degree. Those aspects include experiencing, displaying, controlling, anticipating, relieving and accommodating the emotions of others.

The distinction between males and females is their differing abilities to talk about their emotions. That affects both understanding and appreciating emotional responses—in themselves and in others.

In a crisis, males will discuss their emotions poorly, if at all, because they don't have experience doing so. Why does this matter? For one thing, if you don't articulate emotions then you don't understand them very well and therefore it will be harder for you to deal with them. While emotions are far more complex than words can describe, the process of finding the best words enables you to understand and then to discuss emotions. If you don't have a vocabulary and, therefore, knowledge of your own emotions then you won't be able to help yourself or others deal with this maelstrom of emotions. Experts can help you find that illuminating terminology. Thereby you will understand and be able to place emotions into a manageable context.

Anticipating the ebb and flow of emotions will help you deal with them. That will make you feel less caught up in chaos. That understanding also enables you to establish both *To Do* and *Don't Do* lists for yourself which will further diminish emotional stress all round.

There is no emotional/behavioural protocol or appropriate manner of behaviour per se. Consequently, there is no right or wrong to our individual emotional responses. I suggest that individual differences will be a mix of gender, cultural norms and individual qualities. Anticipate, accept and respect a wide spectrum of reactions. However, explosive emotional release at the wrong time can be highly detrimental to the patient and to the caregiver team. Remove such people immediately from contact with the others and get them the appropriate treatment: rest, a shoulder to cry on, a health care professional or medication.

Stress

As you will have read, the day of the accident we experienced progressive shocks as we proceeded through the events, free falling into despair when the professionals peeled back our son's skull to reveal his rapidly terminating condition. We moved from serious at noon; to grave at 3 p.m.; to doctor-expected-death-at-any-time at 9:30 p.m.

Moving through increasing stages of shock for 9 hours made it impossible to experience normal emotions when the surgeon told us the worst at 9:30. Constructive response is apparently impossible. You are not able to process information and you lose the ability to act. You have been separated from any world you have known. By your inability to respond, you become a stranger to yourself and a useless stranger at that.

This is when I came to live in the *now*, a rolling 10 seconds that was to be my total existence for many months. To look backward from that 10 seconds to what was or forward to what might never-be was to risk puncturing the Sack of Dread that I was now carrying on my shoulders, and carry to this day, almost invisibly.

Perhaps it is obvious that whoever is able to coordinate the care of the others both experiences the pressure and is best able to cope with it. However, they will not avoid having to deal with the stress someway, sometime. Those who bottle it up will suffer consequences through deteriorated health including high blood pressure, heart disease and cancer.

What did I do? Knowing that I was under enormous stress, I monitored my stress levels and took pre-emptive precautions, both regularly and as required. I dampened the energy level, when necessary, by removing myself to a low stimulus environment such as a park, a nearby cathedral, by sitting facing the sun, or walking a nearby street. I talked myself down and did deep breathing. I walked as much as I could. I went out in nature. I added to Facebook. I counselled family and friends. I found counselling soothing; choosing the positive words for others reinforced positive feelings in me. I spoke to Drew. I explored the hospital. You may find your own stress relief in knitting, reading or Sudoku.

Unfortunately I know of only one means to deliberately release unexpected pressure—a controlled detonation. When it arises, I suggest that you remove yourself to a safe distance, and give in until the stress blows itself out.

To date, I had four major stress experiences. I have described the first twenty-four hours when I was either numb or bottling it up. The second, occurred on my front lawn, triggered by my neighbour as I described above in my note to day 4. I nearly lost it but fought hard to control myself as I didn't know if a meltdown then and there would incapacitate me at a time when I was needed. Later the neighbour said that I had looked so absolutely awful that it had put her in shock, preventing her from melting down, fortunately. I don't know how, minutes later, we drove safely back to the hospital. Third, I have described the intense but time-limited Mother's Day meltdown that my wife and I experienced, roughly six weeks after Drew's injury. Fourth, my major meltdown came unexpectedly a distant 22-months after the accident, weeks after Drew had another head surgery when my Sack of Dread punctured at the supper table. I describe it above at page 75.

That stress meltdown was largely physiological, somewhat psychological and partially emotional. I cried. I withdrew from the family, friends and the world for several weeks. I went on vigorous walks two or three or five times a day to bring my stress levels down so that I wouldn't really lose it and need to be hospitalized. I talked to a doctor and I took medication.

None of these four examples do I consider abnormal—for the circumstances. I'm fortunate that they unfolded as they did. I was able to control the pressure when I needed to and to *lose-it* when it was safe to do so.

Surprisingly, pressure still builds for a variety of reasons. Speaking and writing about my experience can build pressure but largely has proven to be cathartic.

Your own crash cocktail might include withdrawal, depression, crying, I-don't-want-to-deal-with-it-anymore, screaming, yelling, throwing things, extreme fatigue, or lack of empathy. If not properly handled, both behaviour and things said that are products of the stress, might be read the wrong way. Unfortunately, they often contribute to breakdown of relationships and families.

Roles and Tasks

I suspect that the role that any father assumes in such a situation is the one that he normally takes on in the family. Fortunately, I was part of an exceptional take-charge family team including my wife, two other adult sons and extended family. We spread the tasks. We backstopped each other.

Like most families, we all could draw on experience gained from relevant life experiences. I've dealt elsewhere with the experience of other family members. I had prior experience with leading teams, with emergencies and with death.

Your single most important task is to protect the injured, and then to protect the others who are vulnerable. Throughout your journey, step up and do what needs doing. Within your capabilities of the moment, assess what you and your family and friends, the caregiver-team, can and cannot do.

I knew I had to ensure that everything possible was done to recover Drew and to protect family and friends even though, in the beginning, I also knew that I did not know what that meant. I knew that in order to protect others, I had to put aside my own emotions, shock and grief as long as possible. To hold my emotions at arm's length, I used my To Do list of mundane but essential tasks, such as dealing with the hospital, the patient's employers, monthly bills, and financial institutions, arranging accommodation and parking, coping with landlords, yards, pets or getting coffee, snacks, meals, the car, pillows, playing cards and magazines.

I don't feel guilty about having deliberately used that To Do list as a crutch/tool. At times I was afraid of the unknowable consequences if my emotions were ever unleashed.

Differing experience and behaviour: male/female, parent, sibling, friend

More than a year after the accident, Neil said to me, "I can't imagine what you went through as a parent." I have no way of comparing what he, a close brother, went through with what I went through. I think that we both experienced to the max. The literature has much analysis and accounts of parental grief for the loss of a child. I may never be able to read it.

Behaviourally, fathers have an experience that is both similar to, and different from, the others. Men want to fix things; and therefore will feel impotent when they are not able to do much. They will have irrational feelings of guilt. They won't have patience and will need to learn that, for brain injuries, patience is an absolute requirement as healing will take as much as a decade to complete. They also need to cope with the fact that some of the patient's emotional and cognitive functions may never be completely restored and that they, the "responsible male" can't fix that.

About this journey, Rachel and I seem to have reversed a key aspect of the traditional female/male archetypes. While briefly we discuss Drew, his current condition, and his arrangements, she does not speak about the journey to me or to anyone else, as best I can tell. I, accompanied by the previously mentioned inner budgie, have become the reverse. From several unpleasant experiences, I have learned to not speak about the journey within her earshot.

I find that talking with someone about your interacting emotions can go in either of two directions: manage them or negotiate them. I think that males will think that they are doing the former when often they are doing the latter. It is part of a larger societal tendency.

Instinct, pragmatic and emotional needs, family dynamics, character, experience and inspiration will all determine our individual emotional reaction. I believe that there is no emotional response template for each family member *type* such as father, sibling, cousin or partner. The only "should" in the equation is that everyone needs to pitch in, to take on some specific responsibilities in order to get the tasks done, and to manage safely our individual and collective emotions.

Fathers' responsibility for the long-term

If I may characterize simply the different primitive relationships that a son has with his mother and his father in such a crisis, I would suggest that the mother represents comfort and security in the present, within arms' reach, whereas the father represents security outside arms' reach, and a means to self-security in the future. In reality, clearly each relationship has degrees of both.

To a certain extent, a father's post-critical-care responsibility to his son is to provide a role model and guidance to self-sufficiency in the world. A father must create his post-injury relationship with his injured son from scratch and it must start with rebuilding himself to take on this role. Rebuilding is very difficult and may never be completed. Together you need to provide yourselves with a cushion of understanding, tolerance, patience, humour and love. For you both, it may require innovative approaches. Listen to the patient, take guidance from them. As an example, I point to my need to dampen down my "contributions" because Drew finds them too much to handle. That requires a big effort on my part and counselling. First, I had to recognize it as a legitimate problem. Second, I had to recognize my need in that behaviour, the inner budgie. Third, I had to make a major adjustment in my *protective* attitude towards Drew. Fourth, I had to *zip it*—my lips.

There may be aspects of the pre-injury relationship that will still be relevant, for good or ill.

A father's responsibility for and to his child will still be relevant but the way the father discharges those responsibilities may be vastly different from the way that they would have been discharged had the injury not occurred. For example, how does a father provide his injured child with understanding, direction, motivation and targets for self-sufficiency? Due to the slow healing of the brain and the need for therapies of many descriptions, you may not even know for years what the new expectations for self-sufficiency should be. To extend the example, if your son is aware of his cognitive shortcomings how do you deal with depression, defeatism, excessive self-expectations, appropriate benchmarks for performance and progress, both in him and in you? Perfection is not possible. Clumsy adjusting is the reality. Mistakes are inevitable.

One example will paint a picture. Even though I worked hard at being non-judgmental, professionally and personally over the years I have been evaluative, measuring performance against what I thought were objective "real world" benchmarks. As Drew began to resemble the old normal more and more, I was reverting to my old reactions/habits. At times like these I had to give myself a reality check.

No matter how experienced I am at hiring, managing and evaluating personnel in a wide variety of positions with a wide variety of expertise, obviously I have no monopoly on knowledge or wisdom and my world is not Drew's world. He has every right to make his way in the world as he sees fit and he has and will do a great job of it.

It was never realistic for me to expect him to fit into the world in the way that I have, to follow in my footsteps, to be mini-me. Unfortunately, being partially aware of that reality didn't stop me from behaving occasionally as if I had all the answers. Why should it be any different now? For the most excellent of all reasons— Drew is in the hands of occupational and psychotherapists who are far better equipped to help him. I need to recast myself as an additional resource—when called on. I'm increasingly more *grise*, but *éminence*—not so much. Solomon's wisdom is but a glimmer over the horizon.

Unfortunately, I found that being *aware* that I need to be a benign advisor did not completely prevent me from behaving badly. From time to time, I allowed my stress levels to rise resulting in behaviour that created conflict with Drew. To resolve our occasional conflicts, we had long respectful and loving discussions—truly—and from these I learned a lot about how insightful and disciplined Drew is, as his therapist had also noted. I tried hard to change my behaviour to fit the new normal but it did not prevent me from exploding from time to time, often at chippy, snarky remarks that Drew made about my habits that annoyed him. At root, it was typical conflict between males, complicated by the circumstances.

Almost 3-years in after one such recent conflict, I apologized to him for a blow-up that was totally my fault. Then half an hour later I said to him, "I have come to the realization that you have healed enough that I no longer need to watch your back. You have the absolute right to run your own life. This realization has taken a huge load off of me." This surprised and pleased Drew.

I meant it—all of it. Do I feel guilty that I made such a decision and declaration in spite of the fact that I knew that Drew had about six more years of brain healing to go through, that his abilities to multi-task or juggle complex options are still degraded? I'm somewhat surprised to say that I didn't feel guilty in the least. I thought then and I think now that overall my decision is best for Drew and for me. It is not completely true what I said about no longer watching his back; I still do and he knows it. However having stated that, I no longer feel compelled to second-guess him to his face, to manipulate by making "suggestions" in the guise of adding options for him to consider. He is healing, he is in control, he is safe, he is disciplined and he knows that should he ever want our active support all he needs to do is ask and we will give it unstintingly and without judgment or comment. Most of all, he will be in the world a long time after I have gone. Even as he heals to an as yet unknown state, he needs to relearn to successfully interact with his world. There is no way that I can learn those lessons for him. There never was.

I realized at the time that this was a major milestone because Drew had *taken* his freedom from me; I hadn't given it to him. This made me very happy because I have always felt that it is healthier for children to earn or take their freedom than it is for parents to give it to them. Drew was strong again! What my declaration to him did was to formally acknowledge a state that already existed and to declare that I would no longer get in his way.

Ironically, it is through Drew's injury that we have been able to be objective about our relationship and that I am truly able to see him as the fiercely independent and unique individual that he is. Even though I have always been blown away by his talent, abilities and personality I am seeing rich new dimensions of him that I had never seen before because our relationship got in the way. Perhaps we are always hardest on our first child, the one who trains us and who forces us out of ourselves.

A week or so after my epiphany and declaration, we entered another conflict when Drew told me emphatically and rudely what to do. I replied, "Just a minute. We have an agreement. I don't tell you what to do and therefore you don't tell me what to do." That seemed to work. He picks up and applies things with great self-discipline.

Things were fine for a few days and then I created an ugly scene for which I apologized multiple times to him and to Rachel. Drew went to work the next day and did not come home for three days, staying with his brother and with friends. I arranged an emergency meeting for Rachel and me with Drew's therapist. She gave us good advice and I met her with Drew a week later. Since then things have occasionally been tense but we have been behaving ourselves and have had no serious conflicts for months. He is relaxing and my stress levels are diminishing. I'm looking forward to a new healthy state between us and believe that eventually our relationship will be better than it has ever been.

All this may sound somewhat like a typical relationship between opinionated strong-willed fathers and sons. However, remember that all of this has taken place while Drew's brain, particularly his frontal lobe, which deals with inhibition and judgment, has not healed and won't heal completely for years. However, his brain seems to be healing faster than mine, which is to be expected since older brains heal far more slowly, if at all. I joke with Drew that soon he will be the caregiver. Perhaps we'll wave to each other as we pass, going in opposite directions.

Patience? Did I mention patience? It isn't easy. There is no road map as such but there are those who can guide you. There will be bumps in the road. But with patience, open mindedness, much love, a sense of humour and forgiveness from you and your loved one, you will work it out. You and your child will grow closer and your love for each other and your mutual admiration will increase dramatically. You will have a deeper and richer relationship. With your child and family enjoy the moment; enjoy each step of progress. Your other interpersonal relationships in the family, community and business will be enhanced dramatically as well. You will have more appropriate priorities. You will see others for who they are, not for who you want them to be. You will be more prepared to accommodate the humanity of others, even if they don't fit your ideal. You will have a better balance between emotions and intellect. You will better manage your expectations of others and of yourself.

Your experience will change you for the better—if you let it

However, did I mention surprises? About 15 months after Drew's injury, he asked me to stop hugging him. "Why?" I asked. "Because you hug me every time I go out, even when I go to work. It's like you don't expect to see me again." I realized that he was right enough; so I stopped. I still get the urge.

Listen to the patient

While this experience-based advice also applies to women, it applies mostly to males, particularly fathers and husbands of patients.

You're a guy. You know what to do and you take charge. Right? Your family, your friends, your society expects you to take charge, to make things better. By now you will have discovered that you can influence but you can no longer control. For some, that will challenge their manhood, their authority, their self-esteem.

You are in a new time dimension that is under the patient's "control". In order to gain any control you will need to make the following major adjustment—listen to the patient. No, LISTEN TO THE PATIENT.

It doesn't make sense does it? Listen harder. Let the patient guide you. You will learn and then you will be better able to help.

There are some exceptionally hard things for guys to do. We are unpractised at *deep listening*—in listening both to tone and to what is NOT said. You must hear what the patient may not be able to articulate. With them, you will need to diminish your presence, your persona. All of this is in order to induce trust, to induce the fragile patient's movement towards you. Making it all the harder is that temporarily you must set aside *your needs*. Get rid of the background noise; your task is equivalent to hearing a spring breeze through the cacophony of a city street.

Ironically, by accepting the need to listen effectively you will become stronger, more powerful and more able to pre-empt and to deal with life's nasty surprises. Moreover, those around you from family to employees to friends will sense that new power and that sensing will positively affect your life. Trust me; I've seen it at work in my family.

When you speak with the patient you will constantly be required to make a judgment about who the patient is that you are talking to at the moment. Always, you need to adjust what you say and how you speak with the patient. Is the mind of the patient that you are speaking with the same as it was yesterday? Or is it the same as several weeks previously or has it healed more? Then you must decide how to describe or position the subject of the discussion in a way that the patient will understand. Then you will also need to learn to have the patient speak about the subject in a way that confirms that they actually understand, in a meaningful way, what you have said. Then you may have to monitor what they do with that information in order to assure yourself that the patient is acting in a way that shows that they do understand it and will act consistently with that understanding. You will learn to easily make this assessment in every discussion that you have with the patient. Fortunately, this demand on you diminishes. As they heal, additional improvements in consistency of comprehension will be spaced further apart. Trying in the beginning, this becomes second nature, a benefit that you then bring discretely to all of your relationships.

Listen to the patient and you will learn wondrous things. Enjoy them. Their lack of inhibition with respect to language and deeds can lead to many rich stories for later telling back to the patient.

Think of the patient as a child. They may be progressing again through childhood, adolescence and maturing into adulthood as has Drew during the three years that he has been living with us. We consider this to be a remarkable opportunity. We are able to help him gain—in and from—each of life's stages, now that we can give him the time that we could not give him when he was the independent-minded eldest of three. In his own words, Drew wants to use this time to make himself even better than he was before. We assist.

He has been meeting at least monthly with his wonderful therapist, Ramona, in order to help him process his progressive understanding of the world, his mental filters at each stage and himself. He knows that her loyalty is to him alone. She is his confidant. She will take his side against his parents if necessary and work with them to help Drew. She helps him to set appropriate targets and to measure his progress without fear or harmful self-criticism. Drew can be very hard on himself.

Learn to see the world as they see it—they gift you with a new window onto the world. You are going along for the ride so you might as well accept it as part of the new normal. For example, Drew's detailed interpretation of the film *Inception* is much richer, deeper and layered than we could appreciate without him. Another example occurred six months after he was injured. Driving, we came across a woodpecker standing in the street facing us. They never stand on the ground. I slowed down but it didn't move. "What the hell!" I said under my breath. Drew observed, "Maybe it is deciding if it still wants to be that bird." Then it flew away and we drove on in silence.

Evaluate but do not judge the patient. Watch their back; attend to their needs—not yours; reflect back the "real" world to them at the appropriate times. They need to relearn what is objectively acceptable behaviour and attitudes.

You will develop new loving relationships with them and with others.

Also, listen to your partner and your family. We start with inadequate coping skills for this situation and need to learn them. Listen to their condition not just their words. Listen with your heart, touch and intuition as well as your ears and eyes.

I listen least well, if at all, when I'm talking. The first major flash point between Drew and me was the pun, specifically, and humour, more generally. While I had been listening to Drew and been guided by him, at some point I became that annoying, hyperactive, jokey guy. It just may have been the result of a sudden burst of relief when I allowed myself to realize that Drew had survived.

I like to think that, in the outside world, some of my puns actually work, even though I readily acknowledge that many are not ready for prime-time. Drew hated them all and told me so forcefully.

Puns require teller and listener to hold two distinct ideas in their minds at the same time. The best puns then induce the realization of a third idea. If it works, laughter follows. This multi-idea-juggling requirement must have been a tremendous challenge to Drew's healing frontal lobe, even precipitating him to panic and self-doubt because he knew that he should be getting the puns, even the bad ones. Drew drives himself to recover. Therefore, it must be very uncomfortable for him to see his father's smiling face as he presents Drew with two dead fish. "I know that dad would not do that. But what does it mean that I'm not getting?"

Compounding our problem was that simultaneously I was compulsively dealing with those internal forces that brought on the *budgies*—my *Tourette-like* episodes. I listened; I tried to self-censor (at great cost, I might add); I improved; I have lapses. We are both recovering.

Occasionally, tantalizingly Drew makes a pun of jaw-dropping quality. I tell him how good his pun is. We laugh together warmly. We share joy far beyond the pun itself—the awe-inspiring marvel of the brain, Drew's brain.

I dream of the day that together we are only concerned that the puns are good, not that they exist at all.

Advice to fathers with injured sons...

In caring for your son, be as good a role model as you can. It is one of *their* gifts to you.

All sons need their father's respect, love and support. The brain-injured need it vastly more. At times they must feel cast adrift in a life boat with no oars. You must provide them with security. Even early on in their injury they are aware of their limitations and, therefore, need your unconditional support. They need it even more as they heal and adjust to their new lives, whatever the *new normal* is. Be patient, wise and true.

Drew's injury gave us a second chance to resolve some of our father/son issues. It is not easy but, with the help of Drew's therapist, Ramona, we have been making substantial progress and have reason to believe that we will put the issues behind us and that our relationship will be all the richer as a result. Also, I like to think that he has made me a better person.

I have always had a tremendous amount of admiration and respect for Drew's personality, creativity and intellectual gifts. As a result of this second chapter in his story, I expect those gifts to enrich my life even more.

But you and I will still want to help. Well, one of the secrets of the light-touch relationship is that in exchange for your loss of absolute direct control you will gain, the infinitely more powerful indirect control—wisdom. It won't happen overnight. Be patient. It's worth it. Take joy in your child's growing independence.

This can't be happening!

You have just been charged with murder.

"How stupid!" you think…. "Who!?" … Wrong! Wrong! Wrong!" "They'll see shortly that they have the wrong person."

But days and weeks go by. You tough it out on your own.

That's false, of course. You call a lawyer because the lawyer has knowledge, expertise, and is an Officer of the Court. Moreover unlike you, the lawyer has the objectivity to bring these assets to bear on your behalf.

So why don't you, one of the severely collaterally damaged, seek professional help—now? Naturally, you have defaulted into the culture of maleness—which isn't working for you anymore—and you are so deeply in shock that you don't know that you need help. The social workers at the hospital can arrange counselling on short notice and your family doctor can recommend others.

You need more help than you can get from the other collaterally damaged—family and friends. A properly trained, objective and experienced clergyman can provide some help. But they can't prescribe medication—if you need it. The best of these will know when your needs exceed their competence and will send you to specialists. Moreover, you need a skilled professional who is not part of your circle because to that objective professional you can let down your guard and stop hiding behind the male bravado. To that professional and privacy-obligated stranger you can safely admit your vulnerabilities, your fears and your feelings of inadequacy. You also need a safe place to cry—a great pressure release that will leave you feeling better. Trust me.

That professional will also provide you with situation-specific critical analysis and technical knowledge about yourself, your family and loved one's medical crisis. This combination of pressure release and knowledge will enable you to re-assume your role and duties in the family.

At the end of your appointments with the specialist, you will put your asbestos jock strap back on and walk back into the now somewhat manageable firestorm.

Major Lessons

From the beginning, accept that the worst has or may happen and then build from there. That may not be the most important lesson, but it is foundational to the survival of the patient, your loved ones, and you. That way you can take joy from small gains rather than be worn down by them. We were grateful for Drew's life that was. That was over. We then became grateful for each moment of Drew's second life.

Apparently this discovery of ours resonates with ancient wisdom in many cultures. Recently, a friend told me that there is a fitting Persian expression, the *Pinglish* version of which he writes is *Dam Raa Ghanimat Beshmaar*. It means "try to enjoy the moment since tomorrow cannot be taken for granted". Apparently this summarises wisdom often referenced in Persian poems, a popular and beautiful one by Omar Khayyam very roughly translates as: *Since the termination of life is absurdity (nothingness), visualize (imagine) that you do not exist at all. Now, because you exist, take advantage of the moment and be joyful.* Other cultures have equivalent expressions.

Survival is not a question

Even though doctors have never told us "Drew will survive", we have not felt any compulsion to ask them. Doctors counselled us about the severity of his injuries, the stages he was going through, and basic precautions to take in his future life such as "avoid head injuries": don't play hockey, ski, or ride bicycles or skateboards.

Before Drew was injured, it was our nature in dealing with most matters to eliminate any between-the-lines uncertainty by demanding statistics, expert judgments and opinions. Then, from our rolling 10 second platform of reality, our new world view saw that self-deluding perspective for what it is: a useful planning tool which, foolishly, we had substituted for reality.

Regardless of the outcome for your loved one, positive things can come from your journey. Your loved one would want it that way. Look for those things and make them happen.

All too often such traumas destroy marriages, families and the lives of the collaterally damaged, particularly if a child patient is involved. Don't allow those things to happen.

Never abdicate your responsibility to the patient

As awful as it sounds, people do abdicate. Do your part; don't give up or be fatalistic. If you are reading this then you are not incapacitated and are capable of constructive action. As you have read above, your efforts with the patient can make a significant difference.

Never rationalize your lack of effort by saying your loved one is in the excellent hands of the medical staff. Never ever leave your loved one's life to fate or faith or to the "Gods". If you have faith, make it an active faith.

In the future, you will want to be able to look in the mirror and into the faces of your loved ones with the certainty that you did your best.

Assume that patients *listen* at all times

Be always mindful that patients in a coma are still plugged into the world and can hear and feel you. Put yourself in their shoes; they are totally confused as to place, time, events and even their orientation in the world in terms such as which way is up, who they are, what they are. They are fighting their way back to the world that they knew. Give them points of orientation. Touch and massage them; kiss them, which engages both their important senses of smell and touch; and talk to them all the time. Play them their favourite music, in ways approved by the staff. Read to the patient messages from their friends. Be repetitive; it may be ad nauseam to you but to them it may be a critical building block of reality that encourages their will to heal and to live.

Be positive, upbeat and encouraging. Do not be negative or argumentative on any subject within their hearing—yes, their hearing.

Do for others

We found that by doing for others brings enormous benefits to you. It makes you feel useful, able to actually do something and it occupies your mind so the Sack of Dread won't. Be aware of the condition, the needs and potential contribution of others at the centre of the crisis. Ask them to do tasks that they are up to, so that they feel useful. Encourage them to support others.

Organize focus for others who grieve. You are at the centre and are doing what you can; others feel helpless, uninformed and lost. Keep them informed. Social media are an invaluable tool to address this; give readers enough but not too much information. They need to know how serious it is but not the horrific details that you now take as normal.

After the first critical 36 hours, set a caregiving schedule that includes sending away members of the core family team of caregivers for whatever time it takes to allow them to recover. Doing so puts their responsibility in perspective and thereby reduces their sense of guilt for taking a break. Schedule the same for yourself. After your break, you will all return to caregiving with less stress and increased energy, perspective and effectiveness.

Accept help

Friends from around the world provided and offered us help, including offers to fly in to be with us and help out.

You won't be able to do many routine things, such as cutting the grass. Left undone, they are a reminder of your exhaustion, hijacked life and the grimness of what you are living. When done by others it will make you feel so much better, even if the tasks are not done to your standards. It is best that others just do these tasks without asking you. You don't have the energy to make those decisions.

Don't be embarrassed or afraid to be vulnerable and to accept help. The patient needs all of your attention and energy. Allow the communities that you are part of to help you help the patient.

Friends do; they don't wait to be asked

Without asking, neighbours got to know our schedule, co-ordinated themselves and left home-cooked meals on our doorstep each night. On the second day, an acquaintance provided us with a supper casserole to feed the seven of us in the hospital. On the third day, one of Drew's colleagues and his wife, arrived with bags of healthy finger foods so that we wouldn't need to leave Drew's side. That colleague had had to attend a critically ill family member in hospital and knew the difficulty in leaving the bedside to eat.

By the end of the first week, one of Drew's acquaintances organized his friends to provide credit with a restaurant delivery service. Drew's ex-girlfriend offered us the use of her condo, the one that we had passed in the ambulance. Later in Drew's recovery on the floor just outside NeuroTrauma ICU she, a chef, by bicycle brought him some spectacular meals, to the envy of patients, visitors, staff and even us. There are numerous other examples.

My brother-in-law, Christian, with whom I was in business, simply took over my responsibilities without asking, but with substantive discussion as time permitted. He and his wife, Marie, did much for us including making daily hospital visits. They also had Rachel move in with them for months, and took care of our small dog in spite of it being initially hostile to their larger, more rambunctious dog.

A business acquaintance at a nearby hotel provided me with inexpensive long-term parking. As it turned out, it came with valet parking. I thought that was an unnecessary perk but I was amazed how important it became at night when leaving the hospital exhausted but still needing to find the energy to drive safely home. The discrete valet team became caring friends who boosted our spirits before we headed out into 40 minutes of heavy traffic.

Strangers will also help. The local parking authority forgave two major parking tickets that I had incurred in front of the hospital in the first few days. The To Whom It May Concern letter from the hospital helped in that regard. Drew's mobile phone provider acted against usual company policy and decreased Drew's monthly rate. When he first got his mobile phone back in the rehabilitation hospital and started running up major charges reconnecting to his friends instead of using the bedside phone for which we were also paying, his mobile phone service provider, Bell, without much discussion reduced his bill by half. This was 3-years before they launched their important *Let's Talk* campaign aimed at reducing the stigma associated with mental illness.

Helping families in crisis to reduce costs is important since, in addition to medical expenses, they will incur thousands of dollars of costs just in travel, telecommunication charges, meals, accommodation and parking and may lose income.

Affirm the patient and caregivers

We found that Drew responded and responds, not surprisingly, to affirmations of life, love, support and progress. Repeatedly, enthusiastically draw to the patient's attention their progress and compliment them. It is a defining part of the accompanyist's job description.

Reliving life's stages

We discovered that Drew progressed along a path that included a brief childhood, and a longer adolescence, with all of the challenges of those stages. Look on the bright side: you get to tweak all those rough edges that you didn't tweak well before—theirs, and yours.

Accept them for who they are at each stage. Don't be judgmental. But also be prepared for the fact that, as patients heal, their mental condition and ability to reason will change many times. You will find that when you are dealing with them you are always adjusting to the version of *them* that is appropriate to the moment: who they were yesterday or today, or the way they will be, or should be. Draw to their attention what, objectively, would be the best relevant decision or attitude. They need and even seek *real world* targets.

When safe to do so, allow them the right to make decisions—and to fail. It is part of learning. That includes access to their bank accounts and credit cards, walking around the block by themselves for the first time, or staying out late with friends. For your own peace of mind and their safety, set boundaries (e.g. a low maximum bank withdrawal or credit card charges), do multiple dry runs in advance, and educate their friends.

As hard as this is for you, remind yourself frequently of what it must be like to be in your loved one's shoes. We are all DNA hard-wired to deal with certainty, uncertainty, short-term survival, and long-term growth. In crisis, automatically we default to certainty. The traumatically injured are in extreme crisis but their trauma prevents them from defaulting to certainty. Panic-inducing is that very thought; perhaps in you too, as in me.

Meltdowns

As we discovered, expect meltdowns to happen to you and to family members. Alert them to the possibility. When they meltdown, let them blow themselves out; don't fight or make them feel or behave worse. If you never learned this before, learn it now—THIS IS NOT ABOUT YOU.

Losing friends

We lost friends. Accept that you too will lose friends for a variety of reasons, which include the following three. Some will be horrified and be unable to cope with you and your misfortune. Some will respond inappropriately. Some will have horrific crises in their own families, from which one of their loved ones has not, or may not, recover.

Assume that no one is at fault. In the case of the latter two categories, blame it on your respective Sacks of Dread.

Those in the first category will just disappear from your life. Those in the second two categories may exit your life either as the result of their decision, or your decision. Others will cope in spite of their own traumas. For unfathomable reasons, you will cope better with some situations than with others.

Friends of mine have lost their children through horrible accidents. In one case, my friend can't talk to me because his adult son died a year after mine was clearly moving towards life. In another case, long-time family friends of several generations had lost a young grandchild through a traffic accident. Rachel and I considered, but could not discuss, whether or not we should attend the funeral. I was concerned that by attending we would be highlighting their loss because of our child's survival; still, I tended towards going. Hours before the funeral, sudden nausea and sweats made me realize that there was absolutely no chance that I could bring myself to walk through the door of the funeral home. This was my reaction even though I had the child that survived. How would I handle these situations if the shoe were on the other foot? Those Sacks of Dread.

Accept gracefully and with understanding and kindness that if those and other friendships are lost forever, it will be unfortunate but "necessary".

Then there are those business acquaintances who, when told of your misfortune, reply with a colloquial version of, "Other than that, how did you enjoy the theatre Mrs. Lincoln?" As a guy, your instinctive internal reaction may surprise you, but externally you will respond in a socially appropriate way. As business acquaintances, such people are supposed to be a business asset. Their inappropriate reaction tells you a great deal about reliability: theirs and their business dealings with you. Treat them accordingly. Eventually they may redeem themselves.

Remember, off-setting these losses will be the many ways that you will gain, as suggested elsewhere. Reflect appropriately on the losses but concentrate on the gains—to pull you through.

Symbol, role model, accompanyists

As we have discovered, you and your core caregivers become attitude and behaviour-shaping social forces, like it or not. The patient, in the longer term, also assumes these "powers" and with them, responsibility. Just as you are accompanying the patient, others look to you to accompany them. They look to you for cues and for guidance. In a sense you become a kind of totemic symbol, as primitive as that may be. This is an aspect of social entrainment. This reality does not automatically confer any degree of positive or negative value. Just be aware that the way you conduct yourself is influential, for good or ill. Use it wisely, for the benefit of all.

Unexpected experiences

You come to learn the routines, the people and the intricate relationships in ICU. You learn meaning; small things enable you to extrapolate, literally, the ebb and flow of life. Weekends were the most peaceful; visitors were strictly curtailed and the weekday hubbub was absent. Weekdays the specialists would attend patients either in ICU or the patients would be wheeled out for equipment-intense testing such as MRIs. The weekday before holidays or weekends, staff would move out patients to make 2 or 3 beds available for the holiday intake of motor vehicle accidents (50%), men under the age of 25 (50%), and alcohol related accident victims (50%).

During my shift on the second Sunday afternoon, a hazy sun illuminated everything through the partially closed Venetian blinds behind the 24 square feet of instruments behind the totally still, sleeping Drew. My exhausted mind wandered as I was about to nod off myself.

Wings beat shadows across the entire large window, slowly rippling across the Venetian blinds. "Archangel St. Michael", I thought, sleepily searching for meaning. I looked back to Drew. Yes, his chest was moving and, yes, the instruments seemed to be nominal. Then I heard the muffled sound of the shadowy rotors of the Emergency Medical Services' helicopter landing on the helipad six stories above us, delivering a critical patient, perhaps for one of those empty beds. A helicopter delivering; not the Archangel taking away.

Why was I not afraid in this momentary larger-than-life experience? For a few seconds I thought it was Saint Michael the Archangel, whose life-sized winged statue I passed many times daily in the lobby but about whom I knew little. It wasn't as if in recent days we would have been surprised by the appearance of an angel. Clearly I was in a relaxed, near-sleep state of mind that would be open to a dream, to an apparition or to Drew's non-bodily presence, as I previously experienced. But, this time, Drew stayed peacefully in his body and me in mine.

After a few seconds did my usually rational self kick in, or was it the sound of helicopter rotors which excluded the fanciful? Was I numb? Or had recent events forced me to be open to, and accepting of, whatever was in store for Drew and for us?

When I went to the lobby not many minutes later, I read the plaque posted adjacent to the sculpture. The winged Archangel is *an inspirational symbol of hope and healing for patients and their families, as well as for those who work and volunteer at Toronto's Urban Angel*.

Did or did not the Archangel pay a call on Drew and me? Was he delivering in another sense? I did not know what to think then and still don't. Certainty matters not, for I am grateful that we were visited by the experience. In its own way it was comforting, ministering hope and healing.

It was not my only remarkable experience on this journey. Expect your own.

Miracles

Fortunately for us all, Drew experienced at least three miracles: surviving the initial trauma and the brain injury; and then recovering so well. Don't demand miracles but work for them and accept them if they come.

Start your preparation now

That may sound ominous or, at the very least, odd. In retrospect, many experiences in our previous lives prepared us well to cope.

We never anticipated these benefits. Our active involvement in a variety of communities, particularly the L'Arche community for intellectually disabled adults, helped us enormously, psychologically, emotionally, spiritually, even linguistically. L'Arche provided us with a core of experienced, supportive friends and professionals.

Many cultures and many faiths incorporate commitment to doing for others. Many also comprehend that by giving to others you gain the most yourself. As we found, giving now will pay off in unimaginable ways, immediately and years down the road, especially should you need support.

Those without caregiving family or friends

In the hospital, you will discover that there are many brain injured who do not have a support network of family or friends either while in the hospital or after discharge. Many others have very few visitors, often because they have been airlifted to that hospital away from their communities. Others may be immigrants with few family members locally or who have been working several jobs and have had no time to build local community relations. Befriend them.

Unfortunately, due to gaps in our health care system and community safety net, the hospitals will discharge those with head injuries before they are healed enough to be able to look after themselves. When discharged from in-patient care, they are still unable to look after their basic needs for food and shelter. They are unable to manage their medications or to follow their out-patient schedules to return for check-ups or for physical, occupational or other therapies. They may have no supportive safety net even though they have years of healing left.

Without any support, often they are forced to live on the street which makes them very vulnerable to re-injury. Clearly this is a downward spiral with only one probable outcome. What our society has yet to recognize is that treating these patients effectively from the beginning is less expensive to our society than repeated critical care. Furthermore, such extended care will return most of these people to being self-sufficient, insightful, caring, productive members of society.

If you are without a personal frame of reference, think of injured professional football and hockey players and the increasingly careful treatment they receive for many months before they return to duty. The military is going through a similar re-think of both major and repeated minor brain injuries. One of Drew's ICU doctors, Andrew Baker, is engaged in such research.

The New Normal

Not only the patient will change. Our other sons, their partners, relatives, my wife and I, perhaps even some of Drew's friends and colleagues, have changed in ways that have strengthened us to handle life's opportunities and challenges. We have become very aware that we are prototyping our lives, moving through each new normal to each fleeting now. Surprisingly, accepting that we will never have a finished version empowers and relaxes us tremendously.

I have become more outgoing but also more insular, self-protective. I try to be more understanding and flexible with others but at the same time I am far less prone to subvert my true self in order to accommodate others, in part because I am less emotionally resilient. I need to enjoy the world more, like my younger self. From time to time, I am more emotional and, if necessary, will *advise* others as to my immediate emotional state. Often I will avoid life's unpleasantness whether that is in the form of people, current affairs, movies, TV shows and even books.

These changes also "enable" me to strongly pre-empt unpleasantness by forceful measures; which can have downsides. These things I won't justify—they just are. They are part of the new now, the new me.

These qualities will evolve with time, healing, self-discipline, the help of loved ones and professionals. I think that I have successfully kept that process more of a hobby than self-absorption.

Recently, Drew has been commenting on aspects of the decline of his ninety-five-year-old grandmother. These include *confabulation*, the use of incorrect words, and the expected problems with an aging memory which seems to return with increasing frequency to distant years. Of course she also has typical short-term memory problems. While we have not discussed it, Drew's observations, analysis and comments seem to suggest that he recognizes and identifies with some of those phases, as if they resonate with some of his own experiences during healing.

His parents' occasional lapses should also give him comfort that when he has them himself it is as a normal part of the human condition and not a worrying personal deficiency.

It gives me comfort to know that as Rachel and I move on into those rearward looking years, that our sons, particularly Drew, will now be very well equipped to recognize, interpret and to deal spectacularly well with our inevitable decline. Our sons will deal with these new normals without fear, with understanding, gently, and with love and humour.

But not just yet. We have many more new normals to enjoy before our normal includes those qualities—more past than present.

On our recent journey with Drew, we've been asked, "What does it mean?" It seems apt to quote the post-coma Drew, "I haven't the faintest idea." Maybe someday we will know. In the meantime, we enjoy life with Drew2 who is becoming not the old Drew but a stronger, different Drew. Thereby, we learn and grow.

Drew Writes

Hi there.

My name's Drew, I'm 32, and I just woke up way too early on a Saturday. I was up late the night before and wanted to sleep in and recover a bit, but somehow my body felt like waking up at 7am. Made some breakfast, nerded out at my computer for a while doing some reading and problem solving, looked outside and noticed there was a fairly nice day beginning. It was early April, just after winter, and all the snow had melted and the temperature was warming up. How about a walk? It could help ease my groggyness.

I put on my shoes, jacket, walked out the door, and woke up in an unfamiliar room. I looked around and realized that this wasn't my bedroom. This wasn't even the loft I lived in. It looked like a hospital room? I checked my body for bandages or tubing and couldn't find anything, so I figured whatever happened couldn't have been too serious... but I had no idea what was going on.

I put my feet on the ground and started walking, a bit slowly, out the door. My room was conveniently located in front of the nurses' station of the floor. As I walked to the desk, two male nurses looked at me with one pointing and saying "Wow, you couldn't even get dressed a week ago!"

I pointed back and said "I'm glad you know that, because I have no idea who you are, or where I am, or what I'm doing here."

After taking that in he replied "Oh! Uh, okay, just let me think what I can say for a second. I've gone through this before, err, not with you, but with others." and his grand summary was:

"You've had a traumatic neural injury and you've been here for about 7 weeks. You were mostly in the Intense Care Unit and weren't able to have many visitors, just your family, brothers, girlfriend and maybe a few friends. Oh, and you've had a craniotomy. Your parents will be able to explain the rest when they get here."

And I thought: Huh..... that's.... kinda cool. I HAVE A GIRLFRIEND!

The last thing I could remember was that I was freshly single. Maybe something happened with a nurse? I figured I would find out eventually, and also I had no idea what a "craniotomy" or "traumatic neural injury" was. If I did, my reaction may have been different but I'm pretty comedic and jovial in nature. It's those qualities which helped me through much of this experience.

I was eventually filled in on some of the details of the previous weeks which had evaporated from memory. I was in a coma, had woken up, was drugged back into one so my body could focus on itself without my mind getting in the way, had lost years of my memory and then it progressively came back. I never remembered what happened, nobody saw anything happen, and all I knew was where I was picked up and the physical condition I was in.

When I asked about my memory suddenly disappearing, the doctors said they didn't know why that happened but it might be beneficial that I don't remember anything. My recovery wasn't entirely pleasant. I should have died, but I didn't. I may have lost mobility, hearing, sight, physical sensation, emotional control, and I retained it all. I had surgeries, I had infections, and I had everyone else's emotional trauma.

Despite all this, I feel quite lucky to be very close to the kind person I was before this incident, both in my body and in my mind. I have some issues, but I see them as "quirks" rather than a disability.

At least I'm still alive.

There's more to my story, but everyone has their own story. If you've had a neural injury, you have a story as well. If you're involved with someone who has been affected by one, then you have a tale in being proxy to their experience.

There are things with my experience I'm going to group into four different areas. This isn't complete, but it should provide a good summary for you about what to expect if the neural injury was recent, or you may empathize with some of this if the injury was some time ago. For the most part, I'm writing this for those who have had a neural injury themselves.

Family

If the injury was sudden and you are unable to communicate, your family will get an insight into your life without you taking part in their discovery. Your friends will contact them for information, and through their interaction and conversations they'll learn more about what you did at work and in your recreational time, how you touched people, and what they cherish about you. My family came to know of my involvement in art and music communities and the roles I played in them. They learned how my workplace took my injury very seriously, and a co-worker even set up a voicemail mailbox for people to leave messages that were recorded and played back to me while I was in a coma.

After waking up from the coma I regressed, to a certain extent, to being a child. I was very simple, could only communicate in small amounts, and I had to be cared for. My parents dealt with this very well, though your parents may still treat you as a child even as you're recovering. Keep in mind they might be correct in some cases. Neural injuries can affect your ability to reflect on yourself in a realistic and balanced way.

Depending on how you are injured, your ability to gauge what you should and should not say to your parents may be quite affected. You may say things you later find inappropriate or just disclose too much information. Your parents may find out more about you than you would normally reveal, and this can especially happen if they're responsible for packing up your living space because you must move elsewhere for your recovery period. They may learn how adventurous you were, that you were into recreational substances, your sexuality or intimacy interests may be different than theirs, or you have a different spiritual belief system than the one you were raised in. Those doors can be opened, and you can discuss it later, hopefully calmly, if need be.

Friends

Shortly after I was injured my family created a Facebook Group (a website tool allowing postings of information and facilitates discussion) as a simple way to let them communicate the progress of my condition which also allowed an easy way to have my friends get in touch with them, and to a certain extent with me. This became filled very rapidly with my friends, but also with others who were interested in what was happening. There were actually more members of this online group following my accident than I had as "Friends" in my Facebook profile. My friends also used this group to help coordinate healing circles among other things. If you think this kind of communication tool could be useful, there are other services often called "listservs" (short for "mailing list servers") or online discussion forums you can use as a way to facilitate news updates to those interested. These tools can allow you to finally reach out to everyone, once you're able to, and say "I'm back! Chill out. I didn't go away."

The local community for the Burning Man Art Festival put together a huge poster containing an image collage of everyone who I interacted with over the years. This gave me something to look at and understand the love being sent my way, as well as images of people in my past who I cared deeply about. They were quite active in communicating with me and spreading updates back to everyone in that community.

Being injured can bring interesting insight into the character of friends in your life. Sometimes this can be with who gets involved, and who doesn't. You shouldn't use it to pass judgement on those who don't get in touch, but it can sometimes be a reflection on their personal character or the closeness of connection to you. Keep in mind it can also just be too much stress for some people to handle because you mean so much to them. They keep their distance so they can retain their sanity.

Life

So, you have a new life! Well, it's the old life you had, now with some "accents" to it.

The one thing I learned to accept very quickly is that life will move very slowly. I didn't go back to work for quite some time. I didn't go out and socialize. I was used to going to music nights and art events, even being a musician or DJ at some, and none of that was going to happen. I had my driver's licence rightfully revoked which made travelling difficult.

I didn't "feel" fatigued and slow, at least in the way I knew how it felt after working and exerting myself. My energy just didn't stay raised for extended periods, and I didn't stick with tasks for a long time. I often took naps in the afternoon. I wouldn't say "I feel tired", but I would express that I felt like "taking it easy". Maybe that's just how I phrased it, but it's important to acknowledge that your injury has a huge impact on your energy level.

Money will be a factor in having an injury no matter how much you have in savings and investments, Long Term Disability coverage, support from government health initiatives, or anything else of financial value. To a certain extent you will need to accept that there are aspects that should be paid for, as unfortunate as it may seem to spend money on some of these things, but these will help you progress back to the same life you once had.

YOU

I still am the person I was. I may have some changes, but I'm the same individual. You are, too.

Often neural injuries will affect your emotional control, or the ability to read emotions and reactions in others. Personally, I sometimes get angry quicker than I used to, but this is something that's easy for me to acknowledge because I'm just not an angry person. When I feel rage coming on, it's an easy "trigger" to help me realize it might be an injury-related reaction and then I can work on ways to accommodate it. Sometimes it's avoidance, just taking myself away from the issue or not reacting to it immediately. Avoidance isn't always productive, so I'm also learning ways to handle the situation and diffuse it. In another way, getting angry is sometimes a legitimate tool which I can make use of. Before, when I would be calm while being pushed around or taken advantage of, I can now react to being mistreated.

One thing to remember is that a large part of answering the question "Who are you?" is the brain in your head. It's who you are as a person and your life comes from it. That part of who you are has potentially, and possibly significantly, been altered. The question going forward may be, "So who are you now?"

Always remember to enjoy the paths you take finding the answer to that new question.

Postscript
Us, We and W5

In spite of what you read about Drew, were you surprised by what Drew wrote and how well he wrote it—only 19 months after his injury? Should you meet him you would be pleasantly surprised yet again.

It wasn't that long ago that medicine's wisdom—based on the science of the time—considered that the injured brain could never recover. Neuroplasticity, then a fanciful theory is now an exciting frontier—discovering and facilitating how the brain remakes itself.

Thirty-eight days after his mortal brain injury Drew said, "I'm not worse, not better; just different."

By different do we look at the then/now difference? If so, which now and what criteria do we use to measure the difference? Or is it best to ignore difference and look at the new person?

So far society has done a poor job, mostly locking up rather than unlocking such individuals' value—personal, social and monetary. What will our society allow Drew's productive future to be? During the remaining 30 years of his theoretically productive life will he be able to actually contribute to his fullest capacity, living a complete, happy and productive life? If he cannot, will we be the reasons? What will we have lost as a result—economically and societally? Multiply that squandering by the many newly brain injured (BI) subtracted from our society every year. Will we, will our society continue to fumble the ball?

You are now inside the BI circle due to circumstances, profession or having read this book. What to do now?

Who: You—of course. There are three yous. There is you the change agent; you the possible BI patient and you who may suddenly have BI family, friends, colleagues or employees. Pull them all together. Be the power of one. Don't let the fact that you will be acting out of self-interest put you off.

If you are not already recruited, is it not in your best interest to act before you are conscripted by the drunk driver, the out-of-control hockey player or the industrial accident? Is it for reasons of self-interest that you will now do something—even something small? You can support those who need it; you can be an example and motivate others. To help you use the power of one, here are some suggestions for you to use with others.

How: How do you—one person—act upon what you now know? Don't worry; the nature of your specific help will flow from your strengths and your opportunities. The opportunities will choose you. Be ready.

Your greatest impact will come from face-to-face telling of positive stories to anyone who will listen. Remember that I stressed the deliberate use of the mirror check on page 97 and the positive Facebook messages? They are analogous to your preparation to become a change agent. You know or have experienced all too well that, for the most part, the injured and the collaterally damaged and their stories of brain injury trauma and mental illness are avoided and shunned by others. Mere awareness splashes on them droplets from the Sack of Dread—reminding them of their own mortality.

Instead you say, "Did you hear about …" and then you recite some of the amazing and inspirational stories from the books by Norman Doidge or Jill Bolte Taylor or Drew." Or you catch their attention by saying, "Did you know that there are 100s of billions of dollars of untapped productivity in North America each year." If they see the positive first then the first-blush awfulness of specific BIs and brain injured families (BIF) will be less fearsome.

Choose the story to suit your audience. Tuck away a few facts and anecdotes for such opportunities. Take inspiration from insightful corporate programs such as Bell Canada's wonderful *Let's Talk* campaign.

Why: If doing the right thing isn't persuasive enough for them then give them these alternative reasons.

You can suggest that they should act now, otherwise when they become the BI, who is going to support them? "Never me", they say? Ask them, "Do you climb a ladder; play contact sports, snowboard or ski; drive, drink and drive; drive when other drivers have been drinking; cycle without a helmet; drive, ride or cross streets while wearing earbuds; or walk down stairs? And your family; do they do any of these things? Have any of them suffered a stroke?"

While they are opened up by that new insight, follow up with your version of, "The BI can be productive in many ways: the old ways and the new ways, some of them quite amazing. Each brain injury costs society a great deal in health care costs and lost productivity from the BI and their families. Lost productivity in North America alone amounts to 100s of billions of dollars per year. Re-engaging the BIs reduces costs, increases GDP, and allows them to contribute and be of value again." This argument provides them, particularly business people, with a defensible rationale that they will feel comfortable discussing with others and therefore they will feel comfortable adopting themselves.

Depending upon who you are talking with you might add, "Doing good contributes many benefits to all aspects of our community—including to business. Others will think more positively about individuals and organizations that are actively supporting all members of society—present and future."

What: Keep concentration on the assets and the potential of the brain injured, not on the differences between then—pre-injury—and the now, that is, shortly after they were injured. That now is ephemeral. Remember the long, slow series of improvements. Explain to them that insurance coverage, for example, at best partially rehabilitates but ultimately warehouses the BIs. That is where there is need of change. In many places, the local health care system does a good job of dealing with the immediate emergency and critical care. Well intentioned families alone are relatively powerless to effect the societal changes that are required.

When: You know the answer to that. The growing concern about military combat and sport BI is raising public awareness but so far it has only focused on prevention and not on post-brain injury objectives and strategies. The time is right. Take advantage of that awareness.

Where: Anywhere is the right where. Use family gatherings, meetings of business associations and associates, your workplace or business, exercise or service clubs, social gatherings and your friends, your hospital, support groups, your religious organization or school and the next homeless street person. The latter needs help whether it is a meal or changes that are more fundamental and lasting.

By passing the power of one to others, you and those you activate will gain immediate and prolonged benefits.

Some facts:

Brain Injured Per Year

In many countries—per million population—4,400 surviving
BI patients are added per year and there are 17,000 total living
Acquired and Traumatic Brain Injury patients.

Brain Injured Families and Cohorts

Based on our experience, I estimate that—per brain injury trauma
patient—there are approximately 180 professionals involved and
70 family, friends and colleagues. That may amount to 31,000
newly affected cohorts each year—per million population.

Social Media

Share your stories

Feel free to share your stories with others by posting them at
www.facebook.com/FromGraveToCradleToNowTheBook

Appendices: To Do List Handout For Family

First Hours

Background: The patient is under the care of medical specialists—round-the-clock. One is dedicated to stay with the patient at all times. However, there are still things that the immediate family can or must do that are important to the well-being of the patient and the family group. The number and nature of items on this immediate To Do list may surprise you.

1. Quiet Room: Ask your hospital administration contact if there is a Quiet Room that can be dedicated to the use of your family for a few days. Both quiet and privacy are intense needs at this time.

2. Shock: Deal with shock in yourself and others. This is a medical necessity. If not dealt with you can't help the patient.

3. 36 hour events: Ask for an explanation of what to expect during the next hours and days, including the patient's condition and what to watch for, what medical support will be provided and any interventions that might be necessary.

4. Bedside support: This is as much about benefiting the family caregivers as it is about the wellbeing of the patient who is intensively monitored by equipment and nursing staff.

    - **Select family members** for the bedside according to two prime criteria: if they need to be there; if they can be a constructive presence.

    - **Schedule family members** to take turns at the bed-side. Start with an hourly rotation. This will vary greatly with situational specifics such as individual stress levels and ability to rest when out of the Intensive Care Unit (ICU). As a rule of thumb, if someone is able to sleep it is best to let them sleep and replace them with someone else at the bedside. That concession will benefit everyone. It is OK for family members to take breaks as necessary and to leave the patient with the professionals.

    - Find out the procedures to gain access to the locked ICU.

    - Find out **hospital ICU rules** concerning the minimum age of visitors, **number of visitors** allowed simultaneously at the bed side—probably two—and **visiting hours**. The rules for critical care patients and ICU are not the same as for the wards and the hospital as a whole.

5. Immediately begin to use **blood harmony** to help your injured loved one. See pages 87 and 103.

6. Primary patient advocate(s): Determine within the family who is/are to be the **primary patient advocate(s)**. Inform the ICU staff and provide basic information: name, relationship to patient, phone numbers. Discuss with the ICU staff or social worker your family support plan and tweak it according to the feedback they provide. Inform your team of the changes.

7. Dependents: Arrange to inform and care for dependents including pets.

8. Hospital Access: Find out the hours when the external hospital doors are locked and the process required in order to enter the hospital at such times. Inform your team of these.

9. Logistics: Find and give to core team the location of washrooms, nearest building entrance and elevators, cafeteria, coffee shop, and lounges on the ICU floor.

10. Sanctuaries: Find and arrange for rest and meeting spaces—hospital provided such as the Quiet Room or local hotels.

11. Outside spokesperson: Identify, ask and brief someone to be your family's contact with the outside world of friends and neighbours. If you can, arrange for a friend—one who is NOT in the core family group—to make the important phone calls to others. This will take a tremendous load off family members who can't handle the task now.

12. Must inform group: Make a list to contact. Assign responsibility for calling or emailing.

13. Succinct Script: For your spokesperson or persons, prepare a succinct script containing, for example:

    • A concise description–e.g. injured, critical, in ICU, in or not in coma, next few days (first 36 hours are critical)

    • Provide cause of injury if you know it and can and feel like disclosing it (don't spread extreme guesses).

    • Tell them that there are to be no visitors in the short term, and no flowers nor gifts.

    • Tell them if you will provide updates via a social networking site. Give them the address if you can or the name by which it will be known, e.g. "<<patient name>> Is In the Hospital".

    • Ask them to phone or to send email to <<contact address>> if they want to be notified of developments.

    • "Now I must get on to other calls. Bye."

Subsequent Days

There are short-term and long-term realities with which you must deal.

Critical Care

I'm using "Critical Care" to refer to the first 36 hours followed by the rest of the period for which the patient will have dedicated 24/7 support of a nurse.

1. Have someone at the patient's bedside when the **doctors' rounds** are done in order to hear the doctors and nurses discuss the update on the patient's condition and changes to medication, treatment and tests. Prepare succinct observations, comments or questions about the medical treatment and give them to the professionals at that time.

2. Keep an eye on the **health of the core members** of the family caregiver-team.

3. Care for the **needs and feelings** of family and friends.

4. Use **social networking** tools such as Facebook to "push" information out to the large group of family and friends. Discuss with core family your accepted rules for writing, vetting, frequency and posting procedures. Discuss the purpose of the site, who will access it, who will be able to contribute to it—including the broader community. Discuss in a specific and a general sense what will and what will NOT be posted to the site. Agree upon the method to create and approve each posted message. To avoid harmful conflict, it is important that key family members have an opportunity to discuss this communications tool, to see its purposes and benefits, and to be assured as to how required privacy and confidentiality (patient and family) can be protected.

5. Use the services of the hospital **social workers** and pastoral care staff.

6. Request an **official letter** from the hospital—To Whom It May Concern (see sample at page 169).

7. Get to know the **hospital routines** and layout.

8. Suspend your idea of what is **normal** and consciously **seek patience** and ensure that others understand this too.

9. Designate the **family member** who will be the primary contact for relatives, friends, neighbours, community (e.g. churches, schools, service clubs, hobby clubs, etc.) and employer or business contacts.

10. Provide the external support team with any special instructions to deal with **children, pets,** house, media (if required), etc.

11. **Distribute this To Do list** to others on the team.

Non-Critical Care

1. Organize **shifts and days off** for all family members, including yourself.

2. Find out the schedule for nursing **shift changes** and **doctors' rounds.** Get the phone number to call for updates once you are sleeping at home again. In our case, the shift changed at 7 AM and by 8 AM we could phone to get an update from the incoming day nurse.

3. Pack and carry a **small bag** with such essentials as an extra set of car keys, coins for vending machines, chargers for cell phones and portable electronics, Kleenex, personal medication, necessary official papers, reading material, toiletries and even a change of clothes. For security reasons, don't leave it with the patient.

4. Updating **social networking** is less frequent but still necessary. If there are no postings in the early stages then people become anxious, rumours will spread and you will receive a lot of calls.

5. Learn about and use the services of the hospital social and pastoral care workers.

6. Find the time and energy to **help others** who might be your loved one's partners, close friends, co-workers, or roommates.

7. **Smile and say hello** to other patients' family members who—like you—are *being there* and *doing that*. It will make both *you* and *them* feel better. Everyone needs a smile and everyone needs empathetic, profoundly understanding friends at such times.

8. Find and take preliminary advice from a lawyer.

For More Information

To do list handouts for family and for support groups

www.marrette.cc/To_Do_Lists.html

Social media Community

www.facebook.com/FromGraveToCradleToNowTheBook

More from Marrette Publishing

www.marrette.cc/publishing.html

To Do List
For Friends,
Neighbors and
Community

1. Put together a team and a network and co-ordinate them. Prepare a contact list with phone numbers and emails addresses and distribute it to everyone.

2. Single primary contact: In consultation with the family, select someone as the primary community contact between the family and the support groups. It should be a close family friend. Get from the family or the social media site their script for the day. Get a house key from the family.

3. Gather the core team together to plan and handle the following tasks.

Urgent and immediate tasks:

- Take care of children of the family and family pets—the family doesn't need any other traumas

- Contact the family's children's schools as appropriate

- Organize the community of friends and neighbours to provide meals according to the family schedule

- Identify and schedule individuals who can occasionally drive family members to and from the hospital. Distraught, exhausted, adrenalin-toxin filled family are not safe drivers and don't need the additional energy drain and stress. On the whole, drivers should listen—not talk. They should NOT ask the family member any non-essential questions.

Tasks that are not immediate:

- Take in mail and papers
- Remove perishables from the fridge
- Take out the garbage and bring in empty bins
- Dust the house
- Cut the grass and weed the garden
- Shovel snow

Set up a schedule for the above items

- Check to make certain the critical items are done.

4. Canvas the network of friends and neighbours as to who might have access to special resources:

   - Social networking expertise to create a site to inform the larger community of friends and to solicit their active support for both the patient and the family

   - Accommodation close to the hospital

   - Accommodation for out-of-town family and visitors

   - Inexpensive parking close to the hospital

   - Meals—restaurants or take-out

   - Lawyers and other experts with appropriate expertise—in case they are required.

For More Information

To do list handouts for family and for support groups
www.marrette.cc/support.html

Social media Community
www.facebook.com/FromGraveToCradleToNowTheBook

Official Letter from the Hospital

(On Hospital Letterhead)

Date

To Whom It May Concern:

This letter is written to confirm that <<patient name>> is an inpatient in the Trauma Neurosurgery ICU at <<hospital name>>. <<patient name>> was admitted on <<date>> for treatment of life threatening injuries.

As of this writing he is unable to attend to his normal affairs.

Please afford this family every consideration during this stressful time.

Sincerely,

Director
Social Work
Trauma, Neurosurgery Unit
<<hospital name>>
<<hospital phone number>>

Resources for Families

Understanding Traumatic Brain Injury

It is probable that your hospital will provide a document similar to this one provided by St. Michael's Hospital. It is an excellent guide for families and friends. Particularly helpful is its explanation, guidance and advice based on the 8 Levels in the *Ranchos Los Amigos Levels of Cognitive Functioning*. It is addresses what to expect and how to interact with the patient at various stages of brain injury recovery. By searching the internet for *Ranchos Los Amigos*, you will find much helpful information.

My Stroke of Insight:
A Brain Scientist's Personal Journey

by Dr. Jill Bolte Taylor http://drjilltaylor.com/index.html

This is a very readable, optimism-generating, unique first person account by Dr. Jill Bolte Taylor is a Harvard-trained and published neuroanatomist who experienced a severe hemorrhage in the left hemisphere of her brain. On the afternoon of this rare form of stroke (AVM), she could not walk, talk, read, write, or recall any of her life. It took eight years for Dr. Jill to completely recover all of her functions and thinking ability. She is the author of the New York Times bestselling memoir My *Stroke of Insight: A Brain Scientist's Personal Journey* (published in 2008 by Viking Penguin). In 2008, Dr. Jill gave a presentation at the TED Conference in Monterey, CA, which has become the most viewed TED Talk of all time. It is available on-line. She was one of TIME Magazine's 100 Most Influential People in the World for 2008.

Community Resources For Individuals and Families Living with the Effects of Brain Injury & Stroke

by Ramona R. Bray, Clinical Psychotherapist Specialization In Trauma & Rehabilitation, A Clinical Member Of The Ontario Society of Psychotherapists (OSP), Diplomate Status, American Academy of Experts in Traumatic Stress, D.A.A.E.T.S.

This manual/comprehensive resource guide is an excellent tool to assist professionals, survivors and families navigate the complex system of brain injury. Other regions may have similar resource guides to this one utilized throughout the Toronto region of Ontario. For copies go to www.ramona-bray.com or email: ramonabray@hotmail.com

The Brain That Changes Itself

by Dr. Norman Doidge www.normandoidge.com

This readable book, and the associated TV shows about individuals with major brain injuries, will diminish your fears and increase your optimism and determination. The central message that you will take away is that the brain can work around brain injuries; the brain can change itself. It is a plastic, living organ that can actually change its own structure and function, even into old age. Arguably the most important breakthrough in neuroscience since scientists first sketched out the brain's basic anatomy, this revolutionary discovery, called *neuroplasticity*, promises to overthrow the centuries-old notion that the brain is fixed and unchanging. The brain is not, as was thought, like a machine, or "hardwired" like a computer. Neuroplasticity not only gives hope to those with mental limitations, or what was thought to be incurable *brain damage*, but expands our understanding of the healthy brain and the resilience of human nature.

Social Media

www.facebook.com/FromGraveToCradleToNowTheBook

www.marrette.cc/publishing.html

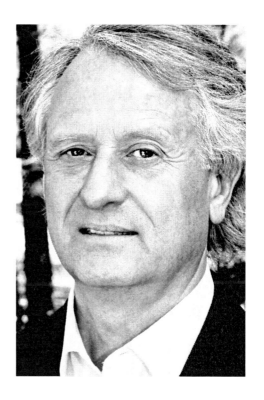

About the Author

Ian Powell has been CEO of various enterprises, entrepreneur, assistant to a federal cabinet minister, management consultant and president of a national practice group for a major international accounting and consulting firm. He has given numerous addresses including to industry, investment and human resources conferences, law and business schools, as well as addressing committees of both Houses of the US Congress.

Ian and Rachel are celebrating their 99 years of parenting.

Table of Contents